Recent Research of Carpal Tunnel Syndrome

Recent Research of Carpal Tunnel Syndrome

Editor

Jorma Ryhänen

MDPI • Basel • Beijing • Wuhan • Barcelona • Belgrade • Manchester • Tokyo • Cluj • Tianjin

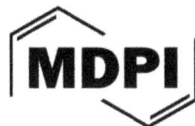

Editor
Jorma Ryhänen
Helsinki University Hospital
Finland

Editorial Office
MDPI
St. Alban-Anlage 66
4052 Basel, Switzerland

This is a reprint of articles from the Special Issue published online in the open access journal *Journal of Clinical Medicine* (ISSN 2077-0383) (available at: https://www.mdpi.com/journal/jcm/special_issues/carpal_tunnel_syndrome).

For citation purposes, cite each article independently as indicated on the article page online and as indicated below:

LastName, A.A.; LastName, B.B.; LastName, C.C. Article Title. *Journal Name* **Year**, *Volume Number*, Page Range.

ISBN 978-3-0365-5799-1 (Hbk)
ISBN 978-3-0365-5800-4 (PDF)

© 2022 by the authors. Articles in this book are Open Access and distributed under the Creative Commons Attribution (CC BY) license, which allows users to download, copy and build upon published articles, as long as the author and publisher are properly credited, which ensures maximum dissemination and a wider impact of our publications.

The book as a whole is distributed by MDPI under the terms and conditions of the Creative Commons license CC BY-NC-ND.

Contents

About the Editor vii

Jorma Ryhänen
Recent Research Provides Significant New Information about Predisposing Factors, Diagnostic Practices, and Treatment of Carpal Tunnel Syndrome
Reprinted from: *J. Clin. Med.* 2022, *11*, 5382, doi:10.3390/jcm11185382 1

Michiro Yamamoto, James Curley and Hitoshi Hirata
Trends in Open vs. Endoscopic Carpal Tunnel Release: A Comprehensive Survey in Japan
Reprinted from: *J. Clin. Med.* 2022, *11*, 4966, doi:10.3390/jcm11174966 5

Lars B. Dahlin, Raquel Perez, Erika Nyman, Malin Zimmerman and Juan Merlo
Carpal Tunnel Syndrome and Ulnar Nerve Entrapment Are Associated with Impaired Psychological Health in Adults as Appraised by Their Increased Use of Psychotropic Medication
Reprinted from: *J. Clin. Med.* 2022, *11*, 3871, doi:10.3390/jcm11133871 15

Bianka Heiling, Leonie I. E. E. Wiedfeld, Nicolle Müller, Niklas J. Kobler, Alexander Grimm, Christof Kloos and Hubertus Axer
Electrodiagnostic Testing and Nerve Ultrasound of the Carpal Tunnel in Patients with Type 2 Diabetes
Reprinted from: *J. Clin. Med.* 2022, *11*, 3374, doi:10.3390/jcm11123374 27

Jae Min Song, Jungyun Kim, Dong-Jin Chae, Jong Bum Park, Yung Jin Lee, Cheol Mog Hwang, Jieun Shin and Mi Jin Hong
Correlation between Electrodiagnostic Study and Imaging Features in Patients with Suspected Carpal Tunnel Syndrome
Reprinted from: *J. Clin. Med.* 2022, *11*, 2808, doi:10.3390/jcm11102808 41

Toru Sasaki, Takafumi Koyama, Tomoyuki Kuroiwa, Akimoto Nimura, Atsushi Okawa, Yoshiaki Wakabayashi and Koji Fujita
Evaluation of the Existing Electrophysiological Severity Classifications in Carpal Tunnel Syndrome
Reprinted from: *J. Clin. Med.* 2022, *11*, 1685, doi:10.3390/jcm11061685 53

Kaisa Lampainen, Rahman Shiri, Juha Auvinen, Jaro Karppinen, Jorma Ryhänen and Sina Hulkkonen
Weight-Related and Personal Risk Factors of Carpal Tunnel Syndrome in the Northern Finland Birth Cohort 1966
Reprinted from: *J. Clin. Med.* 2022, *11*, 1510, doi:10.3390/jcm11061510 63

Luis Matesanz-García, Ferran Cuenca-Martínez, Ana Isabel Simón, David Cecilia, Carlos Goicoechea-García, Josué Fernández-Carnero and Annina B. Schmid
Signs Indicative of Central Sensitization Are Present but Not Associated with the Central Sensitization Inventory in Patients with Focal Nerve Injury
Reprinted from: *J. Clin. Med.* 2022, *11*, 1075, doi:10.3390/jcm11041075 73

Takuro Watanabe, Takafumi Koyama, Eriku Yamada, Akimoto Nimura, Koji Fujita and Yuta Sugiura
The Accuracy of a Screening System for Carpal Tunnel Syndrome Using Hand Drawing
Reprinted from: *J. Clin. Med.* 2021, *10*, 4437, doi:10.3390/jcm10194437 85

Pekka Löppönen, Sina Hulkkonen and Jorma Ryhänen
Proximal Median Nerve Compression in the Differential Diagnosis of Carpal Tunnel Syndrome
Reprinted from: *J. Clin. Med.* **2022**, *11*, 3988, doi:10.3390/jcm11143988 . . . . **97**

Kathryn R. Segal, Alexandria Debasitis and Steven M. Koehler
Optimization of Carpal Tunnel Syndrome Using WALANT Method
Reprinted from: *J. Clin. Med.* **2022**, *11*, 3854, doi:10.3390/jcm11133854 . . . . **113**

About the Editor

Jorma Ryhänen

Jorma Ryhänen is the head of hand surgery at Helsinki University Hospital. He is also an adjunct professor of hand surgery. Dr. Ryhänen received his M.D. degree from The University of Oulu in 1989. He is qualified as a specialist in surgery and later as a specialist in hand surgery (2000). He became a doctor of medical sciences in 1999 (Dr.Med., Ph.D.). Further, he received a position as an adjunct professor of hand surgery (University of Oulu, 2003) and also a position as an adjunct professor of biomaterial engineering (Institute of Biomaterials, Tampere University of Technology, 2004).

Dr. Ryhänen has been a board member of the examiners of qualifications in hand surgery in Finland during the years between 2001–2022. He has been a responsible supervisor of over 20 graduated hand surgery registrars. He has been in charge of hand surgery teaching at University of Oulu (2000-2011) and the University of Kuopio (2004-2009). Since 2017, he has been a responsible person for the teaching of hand surgery and training programs at the University of Helsinki. Significant positions Dr. Ryhänen has held in scientific societies include the Finnish Society for Surgery of the Hand (member 1997-, board member 2000-2006, Chair 2007-2009) and the Finnish Society of Surgery (board member 2006-2009). He is a Finnish delegate of FESSH (Federation of European Societies for Surgery of the Hand). He has been a permanent medical expert in the National Supervisory Authority for Welfare and Health and a permanent medical expert in The Finnish Patient Insurance Centre for several years.

Dr. Ryhänen is a member of the Finnish Medical Association (FMA) and the Finnish Society of Surgery and is a past president of the Finnish Society for Surgery of the Hand (FSSH). He is also a member of the FESSH (European), ASSH (American), and SSSH (Scandinavian) societies. The scientific interests of Dr. Ryhänen are focused around several fields of hand surgery, biomaterials, epidemiology, and artificial intelligence solutions in hand surgery. He has been a writer or co-writer in a tremendous amount of original articles, several books, and other publications in the field.

He has been a supervisor or opponent of several doctoral dissertations and other academic theses.

Dr. Ryhänen has participated in numerous meetings as course chair, faculty, and moderator. He has been an invited lecturer in several countries worldwide and continues to be active as a scientific reviewer (and editor) of various journals. The clinical practice includes every field of hand surgery (trauma and reconstructive surgery, plexus, toe transfers, etc.). Still, his main interest is focusing on hand transplantation surgery, and there is an ongoing project on this in his hospital. Among other duties, Dr. Ryhänen will be the president of the FESSH (Federation of European Societies for Surgery of the Hand) meeting in Helsinki in 2025.

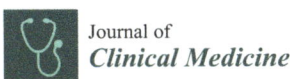

Editorial

Recent Research Provides Significant New Information about Predisposing Factors, Diagnostic Practices, and Treatment of Carpal Tunnel Syndrome

Jorma Ryhänen

Department of Hand Surgery, Helsinki University Hospital, University of Helsinki, FI-00029 Helsinki, Finland; jorma.ryhanen@hus.fi

This current Special Issue of *JCM* will highlight some of the latest studies on carpal tunnel syndrome (CTS). This common upper extremity compression neuropathy can lead to a permanent lack of sensation in the median nerve area of the hand as well as thenar muscle atrophy. In addition to unpleasant symptoms, the disease can lead to incapacity for work, sick leave, and disability.

There are many aspects of CTS that are still unclear. Through active research, we generate a better overall picture of this disease's etiology, risk factors, implications, and effective treatment options.

In the review of Zimmerman et al. [1], the pathophysiological aspects of CTS relating to diabetes are summarized. This comprehensive article combines current data and explains the increased risk of CTS in individuals with diabetes.

One can quickly think that only local wrist-level compression of the median nerve causes problems in CTS, but the picture is more comprehensive. When analyzing psychotropic medication in CTS patients in a large national register study, Dahlin et al. [2] found that surgically treated individuals with a nerve compression disorder have a higher risk of impaired psychological health.

Additionally, one study in this Special Issue states that patients with CTS have signs of changing central pain mechanisms. This might be associated more with psychological factors than central pain processing in people with focal nerve injuries [3].

Some anatomical risk indicators for CTS have been pointed out, such as body mass index, as found in the extensive birth cohort study by Lampainen et al. [4].

The diagnosis of CTS faces some challenges. Diagnosis is usually made from right anamnesis, clinical symptoms, and electromyography (EMG) findings. EMG studies are routinely used as a diagnostic tool of CTS, but these studies also contain sources of uncertainty. In the study of Sasaki et al. [5], a robust negative correlation between sensory nerve conduction velocity and distal motor latency was found, meaning that the severity classifications do not always correctly reveal the severity of CTS.

Ultrasound (US) has also been used as a diagnostic tool for CTS. In the study by Song et al. [6], most electrodiagnostic measurements revealed substantial correlations with roentgenographic and ultrasonography features. The electrodiagnostic severity was also correlated with imaging characteristics and wrist X-rays, and US may help diagnose CTS as a supplement to electrodiagnostic studies.

The article of Heiling et al. [7] concludes that diagnosis of CTS in diabetic patients should mainly be based upon specific anamnestic information and clinical findings. They point out that electrodiagnostic testing and nerve US results must be interpreted carefully, and other factors must be considered.

In the article by Watanabe et al. [8], a specific hand drawing test was used to screen CTS patients, and was found to be effective for this purpose.

The differential diagnosis of CTS to more proximal median nerve problems is essential and should be carefully considered when deciding on the proper treatment. The review

Citation: Ryhänen, J. Recent Research Provides Significant New Information about Predisposing Factors, Diagnostic Practices, and Treatment of Carpal Tunnel Syndrome. *J. Clin. Med.* **2022**, *11*, 5382. https://doi.org/10.3390/jcm11185382

Received: 31 August 2022
Accepted: 8 September 2022
Published: 14 September 2022

Publisher's Note: MDPI stays neutral with regard to jurisdictional claims in published maps and institutional affiliations.

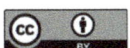

Copyright: © 2022 by the author. Licensee MDPI, Basel, Switzerland. This article is an open access article distributed under the terms and conditions of the Creative Commons Attribution (CC BY) license (https://creativecommons.org/licenses/by/4.0/).

of Löppönen et al. [9] clarifies that proximal median nerve compressions (PMNC) should be seen as a continuum of mild to severe nerve lesions along a branching median nerve, thus producing variable symptoms. The diagnosis should be based on a more thorough understanding of anatomy and clinical examination. In PMNC, intervention should be planned according to each patient's condition. To point out the complexity of causes and symptoms, PMNC should be named proximal median nerve syndrome.

How about the conservative treatment of CTS? In this Special Issue, Karjalainen et al. [10] review the present evidence of non-surgical treatments for CTS. These practices are diverse, and an unambiguously superior method is not clear. They found that many studies propose small short-term advantages of certain treatments, but evidence of their long-term benefits is weak. The article concluded that "research in this area should focus on establishing the value of each treatment instead of comparing various treatments with uncertain benefits".

Surgery is reserved for those patients that do not attain a satisfactory symptom state by non-operative means, but what is the best method?

Segal et al.'s [11] review describes the current practice of carpal tunnel release (CTR) using the wide-awake, local-anesthesia, no-tourniquet (WALANT) technique. This is associated with substantial cost savings and a faster workflow. It can be safely implemented in an outpatient clinic with less use of resources. The authors conclude that WALANT surgery is able to achieve standard or better postoperative pain control and satisfaction for patients.

Another widely discussed technical issue is whether to treat CTR using endoscopic (ECTR) or open methods. Both surgeries are widely utilized, and there are no significant differences in the long-term postoperative results [12]. However, ECTR has certain advantages, such as less scarring and a shorter recovery period. This facilitates an earlier return to daily life activities. However, there are concerns about the potential for transient or permanent nerve injury. In the study of Yamamoto et al. [13], the annual open and endoscopic carpal tunnel release figures of Japan were documented, and their trends, gender differences, age distributions, and regional variations were analyzed. The results show that almost 40,000 CTRs were performed annually in Japan, and open CTR was implemented nearly four times more often than endoscopic CTR.

When the diagnosis and treatment of CTS are too late for the nerves to recover, or there is a surgical complication or failure of initial surgery, there might be a need for some late reconstructive surgeries. These should be performed by experienced hand surgeons. The approach and management of failed CTR are reviewed in the comprehensive article by Pripotnev et al. [14]. These patients can be categorized into persistent, recurrent, and new symptom groups. The operative treatment of revision cases included the proximal exploration of the median nerve, the re-release of the transverse retinaculum and scar, the evaluation of the nerve injury, the treatment of secondary sites of compression, and possible supplementary procedures. In addition, ulnar nerve release with neurolysis in the Guyon's canal is recommended.

Researchers and clinicians from different fields sometimes look at CTS only from their narrow perspective of epidemiology, diagnostics, or surgical treatment. However, it would be useful to have a broader view of the matter. This Special Issue offers an interdisciplinary approach to the CTS problem from different perspectives. I hope the reader will take new inspiration from it for further research, aiming to achieve the best patient care.

Funding: This research received no external funding.

Conflicts of Interest: The author declares no conflict of interest.

References

1. Zimmerman, M.; Gottsäter, A.; Dahlin, L.B. Carpal Tunnel Syndrome and Diabetes—A Comprehensive Review. *J. Clin. Med.* **2022**, *11*, 1674. [CrossRef] [PubMed]
2. Dahlin, L.B.; Perez, R.; Nyman, E.; Zimmerman, M.; Merlo, J. Carpal Tunnel Syndrome and Ulnar Nerve Entrapment Are Associated with Impaired Psychological Health in Adults as Appraised by Their Increased Use of Psychotropic Medication. *J. Clin. Med.* **2022**, *11*, 3871. [CrossRef] [PubMed]

3. Matesanz-García, L.; Cuenca-Martinez, F.; Simon, A.I.; Cecilia, D.; Goicoechea-Garcia, C.; Fernandez-Carnero, J.; Schmid, A.B. Signs Indicative of Central Sensitization Are Present but Not Associated with the Central Sensitization Inventory in Patients with Focal Nerve Injury. *J. Clin. Med.* **2022**, *11*, 1075. [CrossRef] [PubMed]
4. Lampainen, K.; Shiri, R.; Auvinen, J.; Karppinen, J.; Ryhänen, J.; Hulkkonen, S. Weight-Related and Personal Risk Factors of Carpal Tunnel Syndrome in the Northern Finland Birth Cohort 1966. *J. Clin. Med.* **2022**, *11*, 1510. [CrossRef] [PubMed]
5. Sasaki, T.; Koyama, T.; Kuroiwa, T.; Nimura, A.; Okawa, A.; Wakabayashi, Y.; Fujita, K. Evaluation of the Existing Electrophysiological Severity Classifications in Carpal Tunnel Syndrome. *J. Clin. Med.* **2022**, *11*, 1685. [CrossRef] [PubMed]
6. Song, J.M.; Kim, J.; Chae, D.J.; Park, J.B.; Lee, Y.J.; Hwang, C.M.; Shin, J.; Hong, M.J. Correlation between Electrodiagnostic Study and Imaging Features in Patients with Suspected Carpal Tunnel Syndrome. *J. Clin. Med.* **2022**, *11*, 2808. [CrossRef] [PubMed]
7. Heiling, B.; Wiedfeld, L.I.E.E.; Muller, N.; Kobler, N.J.; Grimm, A.; Kloos, C.; Axre, H. Electrodiagnostic Testing and Nerve Ultrasound of the Carpal Tunnel in Patients with Type 2 Diabetes. *J. Clin. Med.* **2022**, *11*, 3374. [CrossRef] [PubMed]
8. Watanabe, T.; Koyama, T.; Yamada, E.; Nimura, A.; Fujita, K.; Sugiura, Y. The Accuracy of a Screening System for Carpal Tunnel Syndrome Using Hand Drawing. *J. Clin. Med.* **2021**, *10*, 4437. [CrossRef] [PubMed]
9. Löppönen, P.; Hulkkonen, S.; Ryhänen, J. Proximal Median Nerve Compression in the Differential Diagnosis of Carpal Tunnel Syndrome. *J. Clin. Med.* **2022**, *11*, 3988. [CrossRef] [PubMed]
10. Karjalainen, T.; Raatikainen, S.; Jaatinen, K.; Lusa, V. Update on Efficacy of Conservative Treatments for Carpal Tunnel Syndrome. *J. Clin. Med.* **2022**, *11*, 950. [CrossRef] [PubMed]
11. Segal, K.R.; Debasitis, A.; Koehler, S.M. Optimization of Carpal Tunnel Syndrome Using WALANT Method. *J. Clin. Med.* **2022**, *11*, 3854. [CrossRef]
12. Atroshi, I.; Hofer, M.; Larsson, G.U.; Ranstam, J. Extended follow-up of a randomized clinical trial of open vs endoscopic release surgery for carpal tunnel syndrome. *JAMA* **2015**, *314*, 1399–1401. [CrossRef] [PubMed]
13. Yamamoto, M.; Curley, J.; Hirata, H. Trends in Open vs. Endoscopic Carpal Tunnel Release: A Comprehensive Survey in Japan. *J. Clin. Med.* **2022**, *11*, 4966. [CrossRef] [PubMed]
14. Pripotnev, S.; MacKinnon, S.E. Revision of Carpal Tunnel Surgery. *J. Clin. Med.* **2022**, *11*, 1386. [CrossRef] [PubMed]

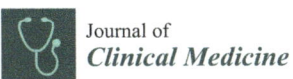

Article

Trends in Open vs. Endoscopic Carpal Tunnel Release: A Comprehensive Survey in Japan

Michiro Yamamoto *, James Curley and Hitoshi Hirata

Department of Hand Surgery, Nagoya University Graduate School of Medicine, 65 Tsurumai-cho, Showa-ku, Nagoya 466-8550, Japan
* Correspondence: michi-ya@med.nagoya-u.ac.jp; Tel.: +81-52-744-2957

Abstract: We analyzed trends in open and endoscopic carpal tunnel release (CTR) from 2014 to 2019 using the National Database of Health Insurance Claims and Specific Health Checkups in Japan (NDB). Japan has a universal health insurance system and more than 95% of all claims are searchable in the NDB open data repository. The results revealed that nearly 40,000 CTRs were performed annually in Japan, and open CTR was performed almost 4 times more often than endoscopic CTR. The crude annual incidence of CTR in the general population among people 20 years of age or older was 32.2 per 100,000. The incidence of open CTR peaked in the 80–84 age range for both males and females. The incidence of endoscopic CTR peaked at 80–84 years in females and at 75–79 years in males. There was a mild correlation coefficient between the endoscopic CTRs and the number of hand surgery specialists by prefecture per population ($r = 0.32$, $p = 0.04$). However, the number of hand surgeons per capita by region and open CTR per capita was not correlated ($r = 0.06$, $p = 0.67$). There were about twice as many outpatient as inpatient surgeries, reflecting a trend toward ambulatory treatment.

Keywords: carpal tunnel syndrome; carpal tunnel release; trends; Japan

Citation: Yamamoto, M.; Curley, J.; Hirata, H. Trends in Open vs. Endoscopic Carpal Tunnel Release: A Comprehensive Survey in Japan. *J. Clin. Med.* **2022**, *11*, 4966. https://doi.org/10.3390/jcm11174966

Academic Editor: Jorma Ryhänen

Received: 23 July 2022
Accepted: 19 August 2022
Published: 24 August 2022

Publisher's Note: MDPI stays neutral with regard to jurisdictional claims in published maps and institutional affiliations.

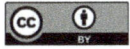

Copyright: © 2022 by the authors. Licensee MDPI, Basel, Switzerland. This article is an open access article distributed under the terms and conditions of the Creative Commons Attribution (CC BY) license (https://creativecommons.org/licenses/by/4.0/).

1. Introduction

Carpal tunnel syndrome (CTS) is the most common compression neuropathy. In the general population, one in five symptomatic individuals can be expected to have CTS based on a clinical and electrophysiological examination [1]. The prevalence of CTS using different case definitions ranges from 2.5 to 11.0% [2]. Open carpal tunnel release (OCTR) and endoscopic carpal tunnel release (ECTR) have been performed for symptomatic patients with successful results after failed conservative treatments such as splinting, medications, and corticosteroid injections [3]. Both procedures are widely utilized and there are no significant differences regarding the long-term postoperative results [4]. Although ECTR has advantages, such as minimal scarring and a shorter recovery period which facilitates an earlier return to activities of daily life, there are concerns about the potential for transient or permanent nerve injury, and these serious consequences should not be underestimated [5]. The transverse carpal ligament is divided in both OCTR and ECTR, although each technique has its own advantages and disadvantages [6]. The regional distribution of hand surgery specialists may also influence differences in surgical procedures, and while general orthopedic surgeons might perform a percentage of OCTR, endoscopic surgery requires more specialized skills.

The overall risk and relative severity of CTS increases with age [7]. Carpal tunnel release (CTR) is widely performed in Japan, which has a rapidly aging population [6]. As the leading super-aged society in the world, Japan serves as a demographic bellwether regarding health conditions associated with advanced age and their treatments. According to reports from the United States and Canada, CTR for the elderly is increasing [7–9]. Being alert to the trends in Japan associated with the age distribution of patients who have undergone CTR will help other countries that are anticipating becoming super-aged societies themselves to be prepared.

The National Database of Health Insurance Claims and Specific Health Checkups of Japan (NDB) is one of the largest, most comprehensive, national-level healthcare data repositories in the world. It is thorough and contains complete datasets of insured medical care delivered within the country's universal healthcare system. Since 2014, this information has been parsed, compiled in spreadsheets, and published annually in NDB Open Data Japan (NDB-ODJ). As a result, more than 95% of ECTR and OCTR claims are accessible in the form of anonymized statistics—for example, surgical type, age, and geographic location—drawn from health insurance claims [10].

The purpose of this study was to document the annual OCTR and ECTR figures within Japan for procedures conducted between 2014 and 2019 and to analyze their trends, gender differences, age distributions, and regional variations based on this comprehensive survey.

2. Materials and Methods

In this study, the designation "NDB" refers to the National Database of Health Insurance Claims and Specific Health Checkups of Japan administered by the Ministry of Health, Labour and Welfare, while "NDB-ODJ" refers to NDB Open Data Japan published as spreadsheets that summarize the claims' data. For 2014–2019, we accessed the NDB-ODJ site and downloaded the following Excel files: "Number of calculations by division, sex, and age group" and "Number of calculations by prefecture" under "operation (code K)" [11–16]. The NDB contains almost all health insurance claims and specific health checkup data associated with the national health insurance system.

In the database, surgical procedures for CTS were classified as either OCTR (K093) or ECTR (K093-2). Information on age, gender, and prefecture was obtained in addition to treatment location, from which a distinction was made between inpatient and outpatient surgeries from 2015 onward.

We characterized the information as follows: (1) *Trends in surgical procedures:* The total number of OCTR and ECTR by year was summarized. Trends and differences, if any, were investigated. (2) *Age distribution by type of surgery and gender:* The mean number of operations from 2014 to 2019 was calculated by surgery type and gender according to age. The age group that underwent surgery most often was investigated. (3) *Age- and sex-specific incidence of OCTR and ECTR:* The crude mean annual incidence of OCTR and ECTR by sex and age from 2014 to 2019 was calculated using a 2019 population estimation summary [17]. The WHO World Standard Population distribution was used to make age-based international comparisons [18]. Calculations using a direct approach were performed to adjust for the age at carpal tunnel release, the Japanese population in 2019, and the crude mean annual incidence of CTR for 6 years. (4) *Number of surgeries by prefecture per population:* The average number of surgeries per 100,000 people in each prefecture from 2014 to 2019 was summarized using a 2019 population estimation summary [17]. The standardized incidence ratio was calculated using the mean cases in each prefecture and the 2019 demographic data [17]. The correlation coefficients between ECTRs or OCTRs and the hand surgery specialists by prefecture per population were analyzed. (5) *Trends in outpatient and inpatient surgeries:* The number of outpatient and inpatient settings by surgical type was compared.

Statistical Analysis

An $m \times n$ contingency table was used to determine the differences between the procedures by year. We used the χ-square test to identify the differences in CTR between men and women and the differences in inpatient and outpatient surgery depending on the procedure used. We examined the correlation coefficients of the number of ECTRs and OCTRs and the hand surgery specialists as of 2022 by prefecture per population using the Pearson correlation coefficient. The statistical analysis was performed using the Statcel2

(OMS Publishing, Saitama, Japan) software add-in for Microsoft Excel (Microsoft 365, Microsoft, Redmond, WA, USA). p values < 0.05 were considered statistically significant.

3. Results

1. Trends in surgical procedures.

The trends in surgical techniques for the 6-year period beginning in 2014 are shown in Figure 1. There was no significant change in the proportion of surgical procedures over the period (p = 0.13). From 2014 to 2019, the ECTR percentages were 28%, 30%, 20%, 21%, 29%, and 30%, respectively, and the overall percentage was 26%.

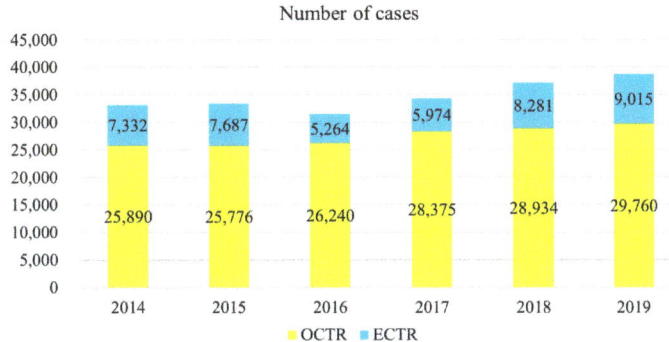

Figure 1. Trends in surgical techniques, 2014–2019 (6 years). OCTR; open carpal tunnel release, ECTR; endoscopic carpal tunnel release.

2. Age distribution by type of surgery and gender.

The mean age distribution by surgical procedure is shown in Figure 2a,b. There was a peak at the 75–79 age range for female patients regardless of the procedure. For male patients, there were peaks at 70–74 years for OCTR and at 65–69 years for ECTR. No difference in CTR was observed for gender (p = 0.99).

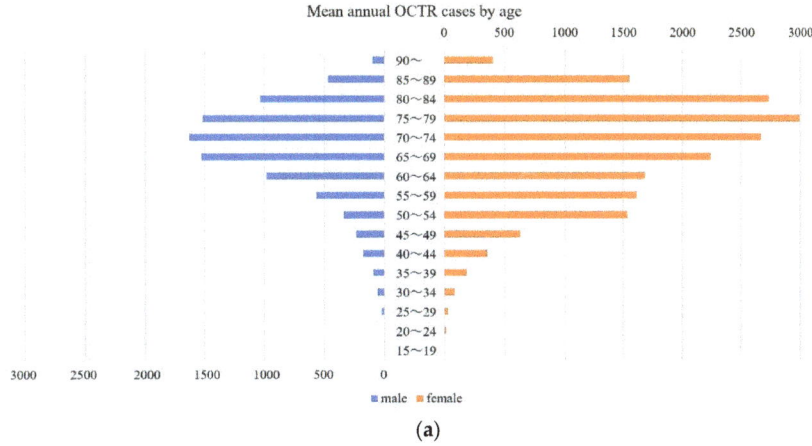

(**a**)

Figure 2. *Cont.*

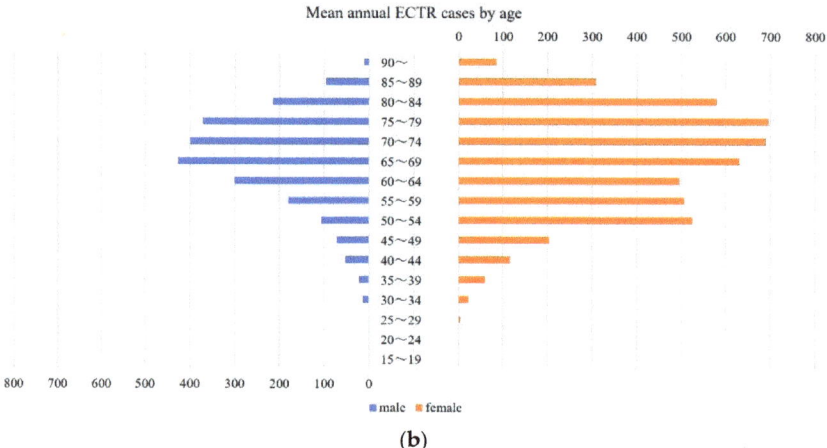

(b)

Figure 2. Mean age distribution by type of surgery and gender. Mean annual open carpal tunnel release (OCTR) (**a**) and endoscopic carpal tunnel release (ECTR) (**b**) cases by age.

3. Age- and sex-specific incidence of OCTR and ECTR.

The crude mean annual incidence of OCTR and ECTR by sex and age from 2014 to 2019 is shown in Figure 3a,b. The incidence of OCTR peaked at the 80–84 age range in both males and females. The overall annual incidence of OCTR in the population over the age of 20 per 100,000 was 17.3 (15.6–19, 95% CI) for males and 34.4 (32.5–36.4, 95% CI) for females. The incidence of ECTR peaked at 80–84 years in females and at 75–79 years in males. The overall annual incidence of ECTR in the population over the age of 20 per 100,000 was 4.5 (3.6–5.4, 95% CI) for males and 9 (7.1–10.9, 95% CI) for females.

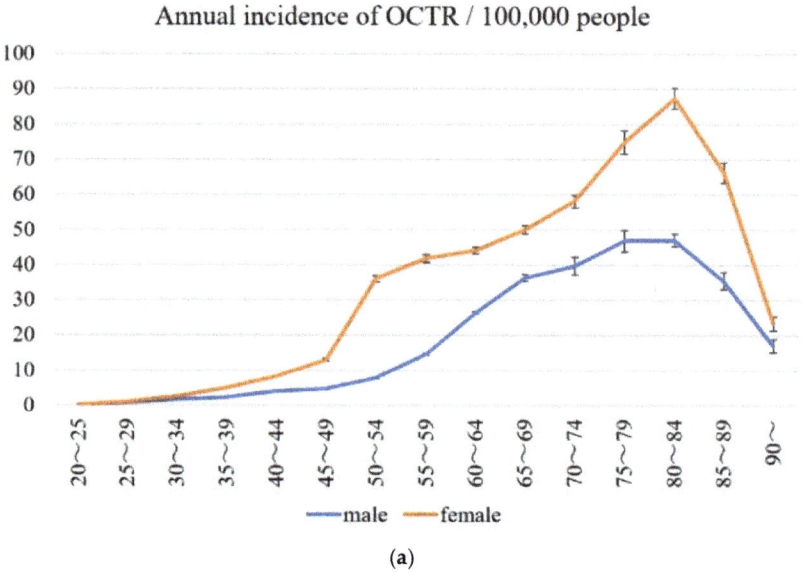

(a)

Figure 3. *Cont.*

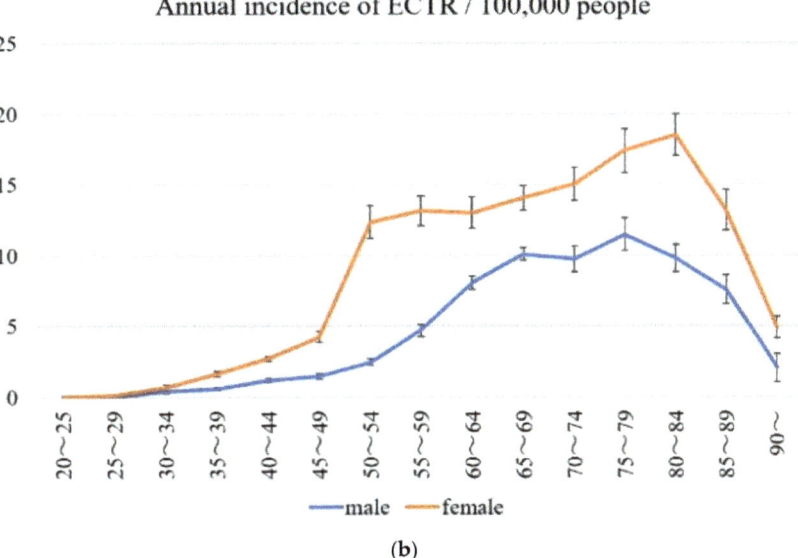

(b)

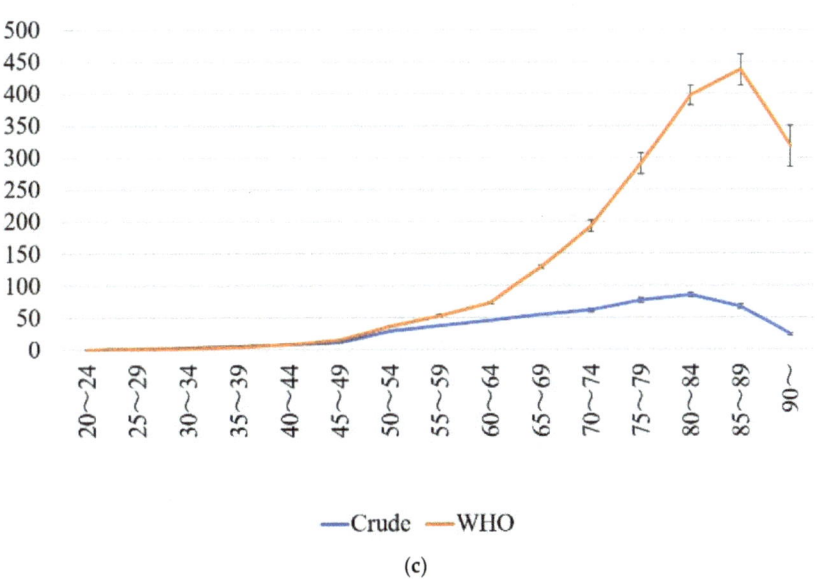

(c)

Figure 3. Annual incidence of OCTR and ECTR. (**a**). Mean annual incidence of OCTR (**a**), ECTR (**b**), and WHO World Standard Population adjustment and crude annual incidence of CTR (**c**) per 100,000 people. OCTR; open carpal tunnel release, ECTR; endoscopic carpal tunnel release, CTR; carpal tunnel release.

The WHO World Standard Population adjustment and the crude annual incidence of CTR per 100,000 people are shown in Figure 3c. The crude total incidence of CTR in the population over the age of 20 per 100,000 was 32.2 (29.6–34.8, 95% CI).

4. Number of surgeries by prefecture per population.

The average number of annual operations from 2014 to 2019 is compared by prefecture in Figure 4. OCTR was performed in Kumamoto and Shimane in more than 50 cases per 100,000 people. This was followed by Oita, Akita, and Nagano. The number of ECTRs was highest in Kochi, Saga, Aomori, and Okayama in that order, each with more than 20 cases per 100,000 people. The age standardized incidence ratio of OCTR was highest in Kumamoto, Shimane, and Oita, while it was highest for ECTR in Kochi, Saga, and Okayama. There was a mild correlation coefficient for ECTRs and the number of hand surgery specialists by prefecture per population ($r = 0.32$, $p = 0.04$). However, the number of hand surgery specialists by prefecture and OCTR per population was not correlated ($r = 0.06$, $p = 0.67$) (Table S1).

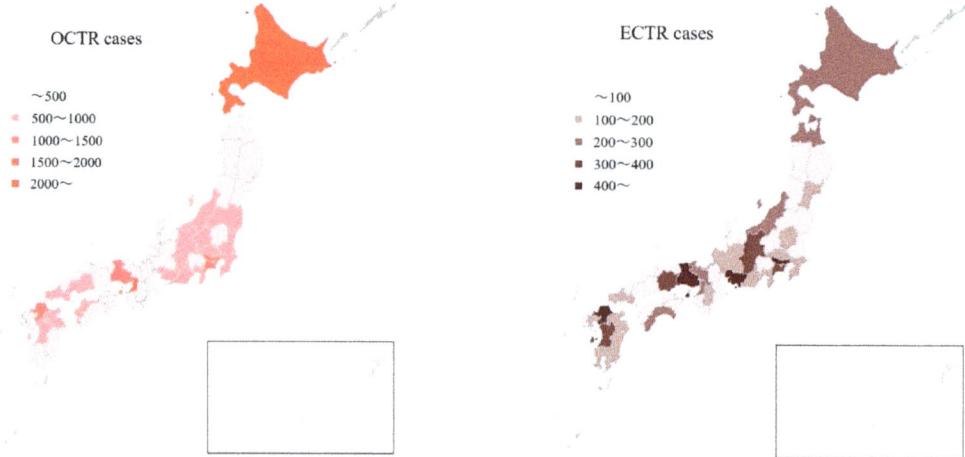

Figure 4. Mean annual open carpal tunnel release (OCTR) and endoscopic carpal tunnel release (ECTR) cases per 100,000 people by prefecture.

5. Trends in outpatient and inpatient surgeries.

The number of outpatient and inpatient surgeries for the 5 years (2015–2019) during which data were collected was compared by the procedure. Outpatient surgery was more common for both. ECTR had a higher proportion of outpatient procedures, but there was no significant difference (Table 1). Concerning outpatient and inpatient surgery, the former increased for both OCTR and ECTR, as shown in Figure 5.

Table 1. Comparison of outpatient and inpatient surgery by surgical procedure, 2015–2019 (5 years).

Setting	OCTR	ECTR	*p* Value
Outpatient	86,972	24,276	0.11
Inpatient	52,112	11,945	

OCTR; open carpal tunnel release, ECTR; endoscopic carpal tunnel release.

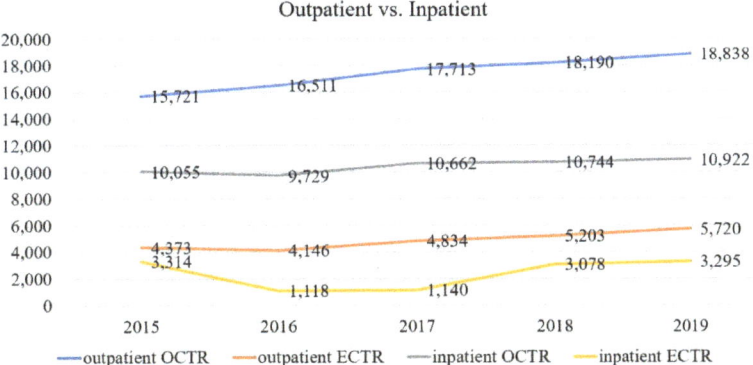

Figure 5. Trends in outpatient and inpatient surgeries, 2015–2019 (5 years). OCTR; open carpal tunnel release, ECTR; endoscopic carpal tunnel release.

4. Discussion

In the analysis of the NDB-ODJ, we found that nearly 40,000 CTRs were performed annually in Japan. According to the Statistics Bureau of Japan, in 2019 [17], among the general population of persons aged 20 years or older, the crude annual incidence of CTR was 32.2 (29.6–34.8, 95% CI) per 100,000. It reflected a smaller incidence of CTR compared to studies from the United States and Canada which showed the average annual incidence to be 100 to 300 per 100,000 [7,8]. As shown in Figure 3c, the WHO World Standard Population adjusted annual incidence of CTR is higher than the crude annual incidence. The WHO World Standard Population has a lower percentage of elderly people compared to the Japanese age distribution [18]. Therefore, the adjusted annual incidence of CTR became higher. In Sweden, the incidence of first-time CTR was reported to be 151 in women and 65 in men per 100,000 [19]. It is not clear why the CTR numbers in Japan are smaller than Europe and the United States. One of the reasons might be that the rate of obesity is much lower in Japan. According to the 2017 OECD Obesity Update, obesity rates of adults in Japan were the lowest (4.2%) among OECD countries. Obesity rates in the United States, Canada, and Sweden were 40% (highest), 28.1%, and 13%, respectively [20]. However, the number of CTS patients in Japan is expected to rise. Accumulating evidence from the present study and elsewhere suggests that longer lifespans and increasing rates of diabetic morbidity are negatively impacting the incidence of CTS [6].

We determined that the ratio of OCTR to ECTR was approximately 3:1 in Japan. This reflects a higher prevalence of ECTR compared to the United States where, according to a nationwide study by Foster et al. of a 5-year period from 2007 to 2011, ECTR was only performed 16.1% of the time, with the majority (83.9%) being OCTR [21]. During the period, while OCTR was predominant, ECTR increased significantly as a share of all procedures from 14.0% to 18.8%. A more recent report drawing upon a large subset within the same database, but extended through 2014, showed that ECTR was performed even less—about 15% of the time. This dataset, from one of the largest private medical insurance companies in the U.S., revealed that the number of both the ECTR and OCTR procedures increased from 2007 to 2014 [22]. In our investigation, there was no significant change in the proportion of surgical procedures between 2014 and 2019.

More female patients aged 75–79 underwent CTR, while the largest percentages of male patients were in the 65–69 range for OCTR and 70–74 for ECTR. Surprisingly, the incidence of OCTR was highest in the range of 80–84 years for both females and males, while for ECTR, the incidence was highest at 80–84 for females and 75–79 for males. The age difference at the time of the surgical procedure was likely associated with the average life expectancy in Japan, which was 87 years for women and 81 years for men in 2019 [23].

Successful outcomes following CTR have been reported even in the elderly, and surgery is performed irrespective of age if it is indicated and desired by the patient [24,25].

In terms of the geographical distribution of surgeries, both OCTR and ECTR were performed more often in rural than in urban areas. The percentage of elderly people in these areas might have had an effect. In fact, Akita, Kochi, and Shimane—the three prefectures with the highest proportions of elderly [26]—had the greatest numbers of surgeries per capita. Even after standardization by age, there was a tendency for OCTR to be performed more often in rural areas. On the other hand, the fact that the number of ECTRs differed by prefecture might have been due to the influence of the surgeons themselves. The number of ECTRs per population can vary considerably due to the proximity, ability, and predilection of surgeons who actively perform endoscopic surgery in the region. There was a mild correlation coefficient between the number of ECTRs and hand surgery specialists by prefecture per population ($r = 0.32$, $p = 0.04$). However, the number of hand surgeons per capita by region and OCTR per capita was not correlated ($r = 0.06$, $p = 0.67$). Reports from Sweden, Italy, and the United States also show regional variation in the number of surgeries per capita, with occupational factors and access to specialist care having a substantial effect [19,27,28].

The ratio of inpatient to outpatient surgeries was about 1:2. ECTR was performed on an outpatient basis more often than OCTR, likely due to it being less surgically invasive. While outpatient surgery is increasingly performed in Japan, the rates are considerably different compared to the United States where, by 2006, more than 99% of CTRs were performed in an ambulatory setting [9]. In Japan, it is not unusual for admission to a hospital to be available for a medical or surgical treatment that might typically be conducted on an outpatient basis in other countries. Comparatively, there is ample capacity—Japan and South Korea lead OECD countries in the number of beds per capita—and the average length of hospitalizations is long [29]. Despite this, healthcare expenditures per GDP are relatively low. With respect to both type and setting, the cost of operative treatment for CTS remains moderate in Japan's tightly regulated medical system, and the outcome is typically favorable. Nevertheless, considering all factors and given the increasing economic pressure, it is worth analyzing and debating whether the continuation of the current trend related to inpatient surgery for CTS remains an effective allocation of limited medical resources.

This study has several limitations. The NDB-ODJ information on which our findings are based did not include statistics on either the treatment results or complications. In the NDB-ODJ, ECTR is identified by a specific code, but OCTR might have been labeled "neurolysis", which has another code (K188) for some conditions such as secondary or recurrent CTS. Nevertheless, this study identifies recent trends in CTR within Japan and serves as a reference point with which to understand and optimize treatments.

In the future, by combining the NDB open data with the medical record information including treatment results, even more comprehensive CTS and CTR trends will be elucidated.

5. Conclusions

We analyzed nationwide trends in open and endoscopic CTR using comprehensive open data maintained by the Ministry of Health, Labour and Welfare of Japan. Nearly 40,000 CTRs are performed annually in Japan, and in recent years, OCTR has been performed as a surgical treatment about three times more frequently than ECTR. The crude annual incidence of CTR was 32.2 (29.6–34.8, 95% CI) per 100,000, which is lower than Europe and the United States. By age group, both men and women underwent surgery most often in their 70s, and the annual incidence of surgery was highest in those who were 80–84 years old. In terms of the population ratio, there was a tendency for surgery to be performed more often in rural areas than in urban areas. During the study period, outpatient surgery increased compared to inpatient surgery, and was approximately twice as common. Nevertheless, inpatient surgery is still relied upon more frequently in Japan than in other countries. The findings from this study will help to develop future healthcare strategies for CTS.

Supplementary Materials: The following supporting information can be downloaded at: https://www.mdpi.com/article/10.3390/jcm11174966/s1, Table S1: Prefectural data.

Author Contributions: Conceptualization, M.Y. and H.H.; methodology, M.Y.; formal analysis, M.Y.; writing—original draft preparation, M.Y.; writing—review and editing, J.C.; supervision, H.H. All authors have read and agreed to the published version of the manuscript.

Funding: This research received no external funding.

Institutional Review Board Statement: Not applicable.

Informed Consent Statement: Not applicable.

Data Availability Statement: Internet links to the Ministry of Health, Labour and Welfare of Japan datasets used in this study are provided in the References section.

Conflicts of Interest: The authors declare no conflict of interest.

References

1. Atroshi, I.; Gummesson, C.; Johnsson, R.; Ornstein, E.; Ranstam, J.; Rosén, I. Prevalence of carpal tunnel syndrome in a general population. *JAMA* **1999**, *282*, 153–158. [CrossRef]
2. Descatha, A.; Dale, A.M.; Franzblau, A.; Coomes, J.; Evanoff, B. Comparison of research case definitions for carpal tunnel syndrome. *Scand. J. Work Environ. Health* **2011**, *37*, 298–306. [CrossRef]
3. Miles, M.R.; Shetty, P.N.; Bhayana, K.; Yousaf, I.S.; Sanghavi, K.K.; Giladi, A.M. Early outcomes of endoscopic versus open carpal tunnel release. *J. Hand Surg.* **2021**, *46*, 868–876. [CrossRef]
4. Atroshi, I.; Hofer, M.; Larsson, G.U.; Ranstam, J. Extended follow-up of a randomized clinical trial of open vs endoscopic release surgery for carpal tunnel syndrome. *JAMA* **2015**, *314*, 1399–1401. [CrossRef] [PubMed]
5. Li, Y.; Luo, W.; Wu, G.; Cui, S.; Zhang, Z.; Gu, X. Open versus endoscopic carpal tunnel release: A systematic review and meta-analysis of randomized controlled trials. *BMC Musculoskelet. Disord.* **2020**, *21*, 272. [CrossRef] [PubMed]
6. Uchiyama, S.; Itsubo, T.; Nakamura, K.; Kato, H.; Yasutomi, T.; Momose, T. Current concepts of carpal tunnel syndrome: Pathophysiology, treatment, and evaluation. *J. Orthop. Sci.* **2010**, *15*, 1–13. [CrossRef] [PubMed]
7. Gelfman, R.; Melton, L.J., 3rd; Yawn, B.P.; Wollan, P.C.; Amadio, P.C.; Stevens, J.C. Long-term trends in carpal tunnel syndrome. *Neurology* **2009**, *72*, 33–41. [CrossRef] [PubMed]
8. Fnais, N.; Gomes, T.; Mahoney, J.; Alissa, S.; Mamdani, M. Temporal trend of carpal tunnel release surgery: A population-based time series analysis. *PLoS ONE* **2014**, *9*, e97499. [CrossRef] [PubMed]
9. Fajardo, M.; Kim, S.H.; Szabo, R.M. Incidence of carpal tunnel release: Trends and implications within the United States ambulatory care setting. *J. Hand Surg.* **2012**, *37*, 1599–1605. [CrossRef] [PubMed]
10. Katano, H.; Ozeki, N.; Kohno, Y.; Nakagawa, Y.; Koga, H.; Watanabe, T.; Jinno, T.; Sekiya, I. Trends in arthroplasty in Japan by a complete survey, 2014–2017. *J. Orthop. Sci.* **2021**, *26*, 812–822. [CrossRef] [PubMed]
11. Ministry of Health, Labour and Welfare. 1st NDB Open Data Japan. 2014. Available online: https://www.mhlw.go.jp/stf/seisakunitsuite/bunya/0000139390.html (accessed on 29 May 2022). (In Japanese)
12. Ministry of Health, Labour and Welfare. 2nd NDB Open Data Japan. 2015. Available online: https://www.mhlw.go.jp/stf/seisakunitsuite/bunya/0000177221.html (accessed on 29 May 2022). (In Japanese)
13. Ministry of Health, Labour and Welfare. 3rd NDB Open Data Japan. 2016. Available online: https://www.mhlw.go.jp/stf/seisakunitsuite/bunya/0000177221_00002.html (accessed on 29 May 2022). (In Japanese)
14. Ministry of Health, Labour and Welfare. 4th NDB Open Data Japan. 2017. Available online: https://www.mhlw.go.jp/stf/seisakunitsuite/bunya/0000177221_00003.html (accessed on 29 May 2022). (In Japanese)
15. Ministry of Health, Labour and Welfare. 5th NDB Open Data Japan. 2018. Available online: https://www.mhlw.go.jp/stf/seisakunitsuite/bunya/0000177221_00008.html (accessed on 29 May 2022). (In Japanese)
16. Ministry of Health, Labour and Welfare. 6th NDB Open Data Japan. 2019. Available online: https://www.mhlw.go.jp/stf/seisakunitsuite/bunya/0000177221_00010.html (accessed on 29 May 2022). (In Japanese)
17. Summary of Population Estimation. 2019 Statistical Data of the Statistics Bureau of Japan, Ministry of Internal Affairs and Communications. Available online: https://www.stat.go.jp/data/jinsui/2019np/index.html (accessed on 29 May 2022). (In Japanese)
18. Ahmad, O.B.; Boschi-Pinto, C.; Lopez, A.D.; Murray, C.J.L.; Lozano, R.; Inoue, M. *Age Standardization of Rates: A New WHO Standard*; World Health Organization: Geneva, Switzerland, 2001.
19. Tadjerbashi, K.; Åkesson, A.; Atroshi, I. Incidence of referred carpal tunnel syndrome and carpal tunnel release surgery in the general population: Increase over time and regional variations. *J. Orthop. Surg.* **2019**, *27*, 1–5. [CrossRef] [PubMed]

20. OECD. Obesity Update 2017. Available online: https://www.oecd.org/health/obesity-update.htm (accessed on 17 July 2022).
21. Foster, B.D.; Sivasundaram, L.; Heckmann, N.; Cohen, J.R.; Pannell, W.C.; Wang, J.C.; Ghiassi, A. Surgical approach and anesthetic modality for carpal tunnel release: A nationwide database study with health care cost implications. *Hand* **2017**, *12*, 162–167. [CrossRef] [PubMed]
22. Devana, S.K.; Jensen, A.R.; Yamaguchi, K.T.; D'Oro, A.; Buser, Z.; Wang, J.C.; Petrigliano, F.A.; Dowd, C. Trends and complications in open versus endoscopic carpal tunnel release in private payer and Medicare patient populations. *Hand* **2019**, *14*, 455–461. [CrossRef] [PubMed]
23. Ministry of Health, Labour and Welfare. Overview of the Life Table. 2019. Available online: https://www.mhlw.go.jp/toukei/saikin/hw/life/life19/dl/life19-02.pdf (accessed on 29 May 2022).
24. Townshend, D.N.; Taylor, P.K.; Gwynne-Jones, D.P. The outcome of carpal tunnel decompression in elderly patients. *J. Hand Surg.* **2005**, *30*, 500–505. [CrossRef] [PubMed]
25. Zhang, D.; Earp, B.E.; Benavent, K.A.; Blazar, P. Long-term outcomes and mortality following carpal tunnel release in patients older than 80 years of age. *World Neurosurg.* **2021**, *151*, e1002–e1006. [CrossRef] [PubMed]
26. Cabinet Office. Aging by Region. 2018. Available online: https://www8.cao.go.jp/kourei/whitepaper/w-2019/html/zenbun/s1_1_4.html (accessed on 29 May 2022). (In Japanese)
27. Mattioli, S.; Baldasseroni, A.; Curti, S.; Cooke, R.M.; Bena, A.; de Giacomi, G.; dell'Omo, M.; Fateh-Moghadam, P.; Melani, C.; Biocca, M.; et al. Incidence rates of in-hospital carpal tunnel syndrome in the general population and possible associations with marital status. *BMC Public Health* **2008**, *8*, 374. [CrossRef] [PubMed]
28. Keller, R.B.; Largay, A.M.; Soule, D.N.; Katz, J.N. Maine Carpal Tunnel Study: Small area variations. *J. Hand Surg.* **1998**, *23*, 692–696. [CrossRef]
29. OECD. Hospital Beds (Indicator). 2022. Available online: https://www.oecd-ilibrary.org/social-issues-migration-health/hospital-beds/indicator/english_0191328e-en (accessed on 12 July 2022).

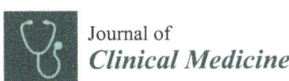

Article

Carpal Tunnel Syndrome and Ulnar Nerve Entrapment Are Associated with Impaired Psychological Health in Adults as Appraised by Their Increased Use of Psychotropic Medication

Lars B. Dahlin [1,2,3,*], Raquel Perez [4], Erika Nyman [3,5], Malin Zimmerman [1,2] and Juan Merlo [4,6]

1. Department of Translational Medicine—Hand Surgery, Lund University, 20502 Malmö, Sweden; malin.zimmerman@med.lu.se
2. Department of Hand Surgery, Skåne University Hospital, 20502 Malmö, Sweden
3. Department of Biomedical and Clinical Sciences, Linköping University, 58183 Linköping, Sweden; erika.nyman@liu.se
4. Unit for Social Epidemiology, Department of Clinical Sciences (Malmö), Faculty of Medicine, Lund University, 20502 Malmö, Sweden; raquel.perez@med.lu.se (R.P.); juan.merlo@med.lu.se (J.M.)
5. Department of Hand Surgery, Plastic Surgery and Burns, Linköping University Hospital, 58183 Linköping, Sweden
6. Center for Primary Health Research, Region Skåne, 20502 Malmö, Sweden
* Correspondence: lars.dahlin@med.lu.se

Citation: Dahlin, L.B.; Perez, R.; Nyman, E.; Zimmerman, M.; Merlo, J. Carpal Tunnel Syndrome and Ulnar Nerve Entrapment Are Associated with Impaired Psychological Health in Adults as Appraised by Their Increased Use of Psychotropic Medication. *J. Clin. Med.* **2022**, *11*, 3871. https://doi.org/10.3390/jcm11133871

Academic Editor: Jorma Ryhänen

Received: 9 May 2022
Accepted: 28 June 2022
Published: 4 July 2022

Publisher's Note: MDPI stays neutral with regard to jurisdictional claims in published maps and institutional affiliations.

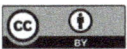

Copyright: © 2022 by the authors. Licensee MDPI, Basel, Switzerland. This article is an open access article distributed under the terms and conditions of the Creative Commons Attribution (CC BY) license (https://creativecommons.org/licenses/by/4.0/).

Abstract: We aimed to study psychological health, as approximated by the use of psychotropic drugs, in a population diagnosed and surgically treated for carpal tunnel syndrome (CTS) or ulnar nerve entrapment (UNE), or both, also considering the demographic and socioeconomic factors of the individuals. Linking data from five large national registers, use of psychotropics (at least one dispensation during the first year after the surgery or the baseline date) was examined in around 5.8 million people 25–80 years old residing in Sweden 2010. Among these individuals, 9728 (0.17%), 890 (0.02%) and 149 (0.00%) were identified as diagnosed and surgically treated for CTS, UNE, or both, respectively. As much as 28%, 34% and 36% in each group, respectively, used psychotropic drugs, compared with 19% in the general population. Regression analyses showed a general higher risk for use of psychotropics related to these nerve compression disorders, to higher age, being a woman, and having low income or low occupational qualification level. Individuals born outside of Sweden had a lower risk. We conclude that surgically treated individuals with a nerve compression disorder have an increased risk of impaired psychological health. Caregivers should be aware of the risk and provide necessary attention.

Keywords: nerve compression; carpal tunnel syndrome; carpal tunnel surgery; ulnar nerve entrapment; cubital tunnel syndrome; psychotropic drugs; psychological health; socioeconomical factors; national quality register

1. Introduction

The two common nerve compression disorders, carpal tunnel syndrome (CTS) and ulnar nerve compression at the elbow or wrist (both here defined and abbreviated as UNE), induce symptoms and disability, which may severely affect the individuals' life, particularly if pain is a major clinical component [1–4]. Nerve compression disorders, such as CTS and UNE, have an incidence of 105–197 and 26–36 per 100,000 person-years, respectively, of whom around 62% and 45%, respectively, are surgically treated [5,6]. Socioeconomic factors have been discussed in the context of the risk of being diagnosed and treated for CTS in particular [7–12], but has been less highlighted for UNE [1,13,14]. More importantly, the recognition and addressing of psychological health early is crucial in decision-making before performing surgery for CTS and UNE [15], and also an important factor to consider during rehabilitation [16], and it may influence return to work after carpal tunnel surgery [17]. The use of psychotropics (i.e., psycholeptics, antidepressants, and psycholeptics and psychoanaleptics in combination) can be considered as a proxy or indicator for impaired psychological health, especially in highly accessible health care systems such as the Swedish system, and can be used to evaluate if a condition is associated with impaired psychological health [18]. Using psychotropic drugs as an indicator of psychological health, it has previously been found that children born with a brachial plexus birth injury have an increased risk of suffering poor psychological health during adolescence [18]. In addition, children born with an orofacial cleft have an increased risk of psychotropic drug use compared to children born only with a cleft lip or cleft palate [19]. Thus, one may hypothesize that even nerve compression disorders, such as CTS and UNE, or the combination of both disorders [20], may have an impact on the use of psychotropic drugs among surgically treated individuals over and above the discussed socioeconomical factors related to nerve compression disorders.

Our aim was to study the risk of impaired psychological health, as approximated by the use of psychotropic drugs, in relation to the existence of diagnoses and surgical treatments for the nerve compression disorders CTS and UNE alone or in combination. When doing so, we also considered the demographical and socioeconomic characteristics of the included surgically treated individuals.

2. Population & Methods

2.1. Databases

The present record linkage study joined data from several registers with individual level information covering the whole population of Sweden. We used data from the registers of the Total Swedish Population (TPR) and the Longitudinal Integration Database for Health Insurance and Labor Market Studies (LISA), administered by Statistics Sweden (www.scb.se/en/, accessed on 1 January 2021), as well as from the National Patient Register (NPR), the Cause of Death Register (CDR) and the Swedish Prescribed Drug Register (SPDR), administered by the National Board of Health and Welfare (www.socialstyrelsen.se/en/, accessed on 1 January 2021). After revision and consent by their own data safety committees and initial approval by the Regional Ethical Committee in South Sweden (#: 2014-856), the Swedish authorities anonymized the registers and delivered them to us. The record linkage was performed by us using a unique anonymized personal identification number.

The SPDR contains information about all drug dispensations in the Swedish pharmacies, except from stockpiles in nursing homes and hospital wards, coded according to the Anatomical Therapeutic Chemical (ATC) classification system, while the NPR codes discharge diagnoses from hospital and outpatient clinics according to the International Classification of Diseases and Causes of Death, 10th version (ICD-10). The NPR also records and codes clinical and surgical procedures according to the Swedish Classification of Care Procedures (SCCP). The TPR and the LISA database provide demographic and socioeconomic information.

Our research database consisted of the total Swedish population of 2010 (i.e., residing in Sweden 31 December 2010). From the approximately 9.4 million people, we excluded those who died (n = 95,618) or emigrated (n = 49,939) during the one year follow up, individuals residing less than five years in the country (n = 423,414), those whose sex was not registered (n = 335) and people without information on country of birth (COB) (n = 60,564). We also excluded people below the age of 25 years and above the age of 80 (n = 3,027,306). In addition, we excluded those with previous CTS-UNE operation (n = 12,250). The final sample consisted of around 5.8 million people (Figure 1).

2.2. Assessment of Variables

We defined nerve compression disorders according to the ICD-10 and SCCP codes simultaneously registered at the hospital discharge as *surgery for carpal tunnel syndrome* (CTS) (ICD-10: G56.0 and SCCP: ACC51) and *surgery for ulnar nerve compression at the elbow or wrist* (both here defined and abbreviated as UNE) (ICD-10: G56.2 and SCCP: ACC53). In the analyses, we distinguished between CTS, UNE or both CTS and UNE if the hospital discharge simultaneously presented both diagnoses and surgical procedures.

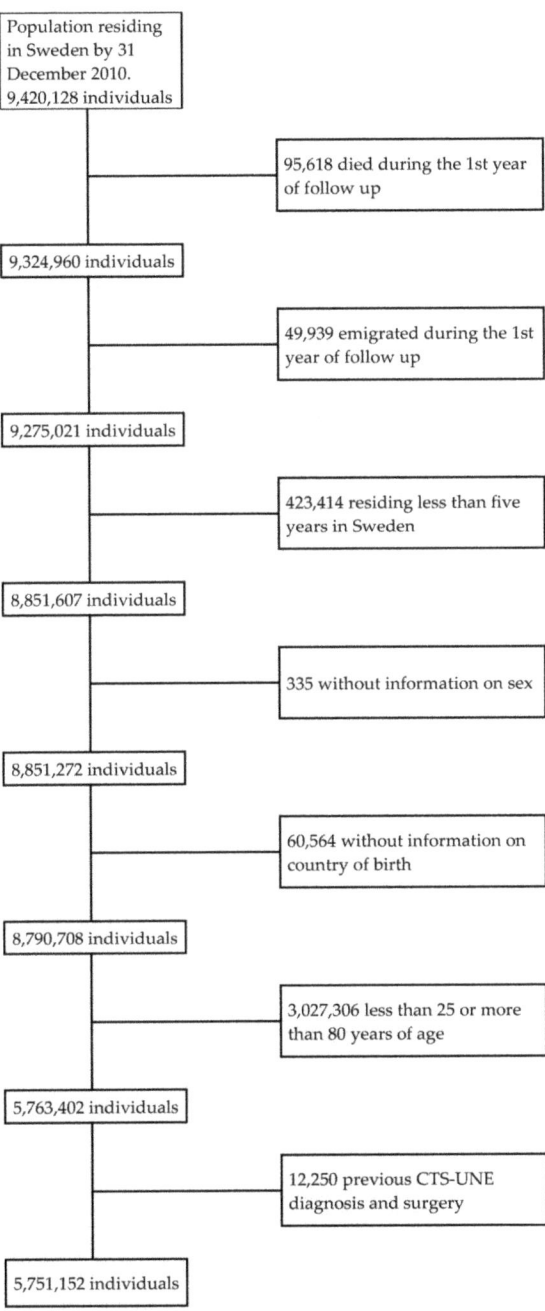

Figure 1. Flow chart showing the individuals excluded from the original 2010 Swedish population to obtain the final study sample.

We assigned an individual baseline date to every individual, defined by the date of the first CTS/UNE diagnosis in 2011, or 1 January 2011 if the individual did not have any CTS/UNE diagnosis. Thereafter, we followed everyone for one year from the baseline date (the follow-up could extend until 31 December 2012) in order to ascertain their use of psychotropics defined as at least one dispensation (ATC code) of Psycholeptics (N05), Antidepressants (N06A) or Psycholeptics and Psychoanaleptics in combination (N06C). We considered use of psychotropics as a proxy for impaired psychological health as discussed elsewhere [18].

Previous psychotropic drug use defined at any dispensation of Psycholeptics (N05), Antidepressant (N06A) or Psycholeptics and Psychoanaleptics in combination (N06C) five years before the baseline.

Age was arbitrarily classed into five wide categories, i.e., 25–34 (reference), 35–44, 45–54, 55–64 and 65–80 year-olds. In age-stratified regression analyses, we included continuous age as a quadratic function. We used essentially ten-year categories for descriptive purposes in Figure 2 (25–34, 35–44, 45–54, 55–64 and 65–80 year-olds). Sex was coded as male (reference) or female according to the register. We categorized the individuals according to their COB as born in Sweden (reference) or not (i.e., immigrant). We obtained information on individualized disposable family income for the years 2000, 2005 and 2010 to compute a cumulative measure that considers the size of the household and the consumption weight of the individuals according to Statistics Sweden. For each of the three years, income levels were categorized into 25 groups (1–25) by quantiles using the complete Swedish population. These groups from the respective three years were summed up, so that everyone received a value between 3 (always in the lowest income group) and 75 (always in the highest income group). We categorized this cumulative income into three groups by tertiles [low, medium or high (reference) income]. Individuals with missing values on income during 2000 or 2005 were assigned the values for the year 2010. No individuals had missing income data for 2010.

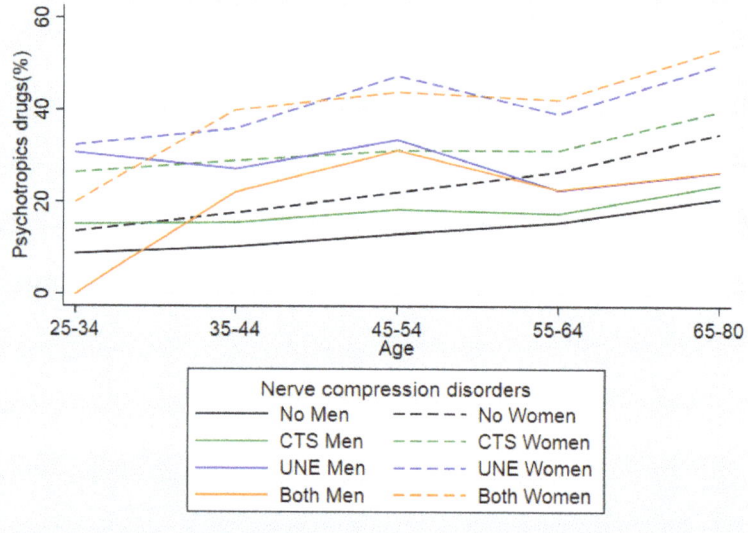

Figure 2. Age stratified percentage of use of psychotropic drugs in men and in women, residing in Sweden 2010, and suffering from carpal tunnel syndrome (CTS), ulnar nerve entrapment (UNE) and both disorders as well as in people without any nerve compression disorder.

Occupational qualification level was categorized into five skill groups, which reflect the type of working task and their complexity (low, middle-low, middle-high, high, and missing) according to the Swedish Standard Classification of Occupations 2012 [21]. The major groups in SSYK2012 are associated with the following skill levels: managers, commissioned officers and occupation requiring advanced level of higher education were classified as high level; occupation managers in service industries, occupations requiring higher education qualifications or equivalent and non-commissioned officers were classified as middle-high; administration and customer service clerks, service, care and shop sales workers, agricultural, horticultural, forestry and fishery workers, building and manufacturing and transport workers and manufacturing and transport workers were classified as middle–low; elementary occupation was classified as low level. If no information was available [553,865 individuals (9.61%)], the case was classified as missing. The distribution of age in cases with no information in occupation was 15.9% between 25 and 34 years old, 13.2% between 35 and 44, 17.4% between 45 and 54, 24.1% between 55 and 64 and 29.5% 65 or more years old.

2.3. Statistical Analyses

We performed age-stratified analyses to calculate the absolute risk (AR), the absolute risk difference (ARD) and 95% confidence intervals of use of psychotropics in relation to the existence of the nerve compression disorders.

Since prevalence of the outcomes was relatively high, we measured the relative associations between the explanatory variables and use of psychoactive drugs by prevalence ratios (PRs) rather than by odds ratios [22]. For this purpose, we applied Cox proportional hazards regression models with a constant follow-up time equal to 1. We developed two regression models. Model 1 included only the nerve compression disorders and model 2 added socioeconomic and demographic variables (i.e., age, sex, income, country of birth and occupational qualification level).

We estimated the discriminatory accuracy (DA) for each model by calculating the area under the receiver operating characteristic curve (AUC) and its 95% confidence intervals (CI). The value of the AUC ranges from 0.5 to 1, with 1 representing perfect discrimination and 0.5 indicating no predictive accuracy [23]. Using the criteria proposed by Hosmer and Lemeshow [24], we classified DA as absent or very weak (AUC = 0.5–0.6), poor (AUC >0.6–$\leq$ 0.7), acceptable (AUC > 0.7–$\leq$ 0.8) or excellent (AUC > 0.8–0.90) and outstanding (AUC > 0–90).

3. Results

3.1. Demographic and Socioeconomic Characteristics of the Population

The characteristics of the surgically treated individuals with the actual nerve compression disorders, CTS, UNE or both, residing in Sweden by 2010 and included in the study, are presented in Table 1. Among the 5.8 million individuals 25–80 years old, 9728 (0.17%) individuals had CTS, 890 (0.02%) individuals had UNE and in addition 149 (0.00%) individuals were surgically treated for a diagnosis of both CTS and UNE.

Table 1. Characteristics of the 5,751,152 individuals residing in Sweden by 2010 and included in the study sample in relation to the existence of diagnosed and surgically treated carpal tunnel syndrome (CTS), ulnar nerve entrapment (UNE), or both by use of psychotropic drugs as well as demographical and socioeconomic factors. Values are number and percentages (%).

	Nerve Compression Disorders			
	None	CTS	UNE	Both
Study sample	5,740,385 (99.81)	9728 (0.17)	890 (0.02)	149 (0.00)
Psychotropic drugs	1,072,677 (18.69)	2,732 (28.08)	305 (34.27)	53 (35.57)
Age (years)				
25–34	997,168 (17.37)	803 (8.25)	73 (8.20)	6 (4.03)
35–44	1,183,624 (20.62)	1689 (17.36)	188 (21.12)	24 (16.11)
45–54	1,165,714 (20.31)	2522 (25.93)	260 (29.21)	41 (27.52)
55–64	1,147,095 (19.98)	2205 (22.67)	234 (26.29)	41 (32.21)
65–80	1,246,784 (21.72)	2509 (25.79)	135 (15.17)	30 (20.13)
Men	2,865,465 (49.92)	3149 (32.37)	483 (54.27)	63 (42.28)
Income				
Low	1,309,528 (22.81)	2520 (25.90)	236 (26.52)	31 (20.81)
Middle	2,038,179 (35.51)	3646 (37.48)	351 (39.44)	57 (38.26)
High	2,392,678 (41.68)	3562 (36.62)	303 (34.04)	61 (40.94)
Immigrant	778,468 (13.56)	1150 (11.82)	118 (13.26)	24 (16.11)
Occupational qualification level				
Low	329,645 (5.74)	804 (8.26)	68 (7.64)	15 (10.07)
Middle-low	2,611,706 (45.50)	5469 (56.22)	525 (58.99)	73 (48.99)
Middle-high	980,117 (17.07)	1300 (13.36)	94 (10.56)	28 (18.79)
High	1,267,169 (22.07)	1326 (13.63)	115 (12.92)	18 (12.08)
Missing	551,748 (9.61)	829 (8.52)	88 (9.4889)	15 (10.07)
Previous psychotropic use	1,608,486 (28.02)	3993 (41.05)	440 (49.44)	80 (53.69)

The age distribution of the nerve compression disorders showed a slight increase of CTS with age and with a peak between 45 and 54 years of age (Table 1). Overall, there were more women than men among individuals with CTS and among individuals with both CTS and UNE, while the sex distribution was equal among the individuals with UNE (Table 1). Compared with the group with no nerve compression disorders, there were essentially small differences in the distribution of income, but high-income individuals were underrepresented and low-income overrepresented in the groups with the three different nerve compression disorders (Table 1). The number of immigrants with diagnosed and surgically treated nerve compression disorders was lower, but proportionally rather similar across the nerve compression disorder categories. The occupational qualification levels showed a difference with higher proportions of individuals with low and middle low qualification levels in individuals with nerve compression disorders. In accordance, the proportions were lower among individuals with middle-high and high qualifications. Missing information on occupational qualification level was rather similarly distributed across the categories of nerve compression disorders (Table 1).

3.2. Use of Psychotropic Medication

Of the adults diagnosed with CTS, UNE and both disorders, 28%, 34% and 36%, respectively, used psychotropic drugs, while this proportion was only 19% in the adult general population (Table 1). The use of psychotropic drugs across the age groups, divided by sex and the three different nerve compression disorders are presented in Figure 2. Overall, women had a higher use of psychotropic drugs than men and there were higher proportions of use of psychotropic drugs among surgically treated individuals with nerve compression disorders than among individuals without such disorders across all age categories except for men older than 54 years.

We used two different regression models to analyze the use of psychotropic drugs (Table 2). In the first model, including only the nerve compression disorders, there was an increased risk for the use of psychotropic drugs compared to the individuals without nerve compression disorders. In relative terms, this increased risk was lower in individuals with CTS (Prevalence Ratio; PR = 1.50) than in individuals with UNE (PR = 1.83) or with the combination of both the nerve compression disorders (PR = 1.90). In the second model including age, sex, income, occupational qualification level, COB and previous psychotropic use. The adjusted PRs of the nerve compression disorders were reduced but remained conclusively high. Higher age, being a woman, having a low income and a low occupational qualification level increased the risk for use of psychotropic drugs (Table 2). Being born outside Sweden showed a slight, but non-significant, lower risk for use of psychotropic drugs. As expected, previous use of psychotropic medication was strongly associated with psychotropic use after the operation. (PR = 15.59).

Table 3 shows age stratified unadjusted AR and ARD of psychotropic medication use during 2010 in relation to CTS, UNE, or both in the 5,751,152 individuals aged 25–80 years residing in Sweden by 2010. The unadjusted AR of psychotropic medication use was higher in all the categories of nerve compression disorders than in the general population without such disorders, except for in the oldest age group with both diagnoses. Overall, the ARD was systematically higher in the three categories of the surgically treated individuals with the nerve compression disorder than in those without such a diagnosis (Table 3). However, the 95% CI showed a large uncertainty in elderly individuals with UNE or both CTS-UNE categories.

Table 2. Crude (Model 1) and adjusted (Model 2) for demographical and socioeconomic factors association between the existence of diagnosed and surgically treated carpal tunnel syndrome (CTS), ulnar nerve entrapment (UNE), or both and use of psychotropic drugs during the follow-up in the 5,751,152 individuals aged 25–80 residing in Sweden by 2010. Values are prevalence ratios (PR) and 95% confidence intervals (CI).

	Model 1	Model 2
	PR (95% CI)	PR (95% CI)
Nerve compression disorders		
• None	Ref	Ref
• CTS	1.50 (1.45–1.56)	1.06 (1.02–1.10)
• UNE	1.83 (1.64–2.05)	1.16 (1.04–1.29)
• Both	1.90 (1.45–2.49)	1.08 (0.83–1.42)
Age (years)		
• 25–34		Ref
• 35–44		1.12 (1.11–1.13)
• 45–54		1.20 (1.19–1.21)
• 55–64		1.30 (1.29–1.31)
• 65–80		1.49 (1.48–1.50)
Men		Ref
• Women		1.15 (1.15–1.16)
Income		
• Low		1.07 (1.07–1.08)
• Middle		1.07 (1.06–1.07)
• High		Ref
Native		Ref
• Immigrants		0.89 (0.89–0.90)
Occupational qualification level		
• Low		1.06 (1.05–1.07)
• Middle-low		1.04 (1.03–1.04)
• Middle-high		1.00 (1.00–1.01)
• High		Ref
• Missing		1.27 (1.26–1.42)
Previous psychotropic drugs use		
• Yes		15.59 (15.50–15.67)
AUC	0.501	0.885

Table 3. Age stratified unadjusted absolute risk (AR), absolute risk difference (ARD) and 95% confidence intervals (CI) of psychotropic medication use during the follow-up in relation to the existence of diagnosed and surgically treated carpal tunnel syndrome (CTS), ulnar nerve entrapment (UNE), or both in the 5,751,152 individuals aged 25–80 years residing in Sweden by 2010.

	Nerve Compression Disorders											
Age (Years)	None			CTS			UNE			Both		
	N	AR	ARD	N	AR	ARD (95% CI)	N	AR	ARD (95% CI)	N	AR	ARD (95% CI)
25–34	997,168	11.09	Ref.	803	23.66	12.57 (9.63–15.51)	73	31.51	20.42 (9.76–31.07)	6	16.67	5.58 (−24.24–35.40)
35–44	1,183,624	13.90	Ref	1689	25.46	11.55 (9.48–13.36)	188	31.92	18.01 (11.35–24.68)	24	33.33	19.43 (0.57–38.29)
45–54	1,162,714	17.54	Ref	2522	27.87	10.33 (8.25–12.09)	260	40.00	22.46 (16.50–28.41)	41	39.02	21.48 (6.55–34.42)
55–64	1,147,095	21.10	Ref	2205	26.49	5.39 (3.54–7.23)	234	29.49	8.39 (2.55–14.23)	48	33.33	12.24 (−1.10–25.57)
65–80	1,246,784	28.15	Ref	2509	32.88	4.73 (2.89–6.57)	135	36.30	8.15 (0.03–16.26)	30	40.01	11.85 (−5.68–29.38)

4. Discussion

The present age stratified analysis of 5.8 million individuals, 25–80 years and residing at least five years in Sweden by 2010, provides observational evidence of the existence of impaired psychological health after surgery for the two common nerve compression disorders, CTS and UNE, or for a combination of the two conditions. The use of psychotropic drugs can be considered as an indicator for impaired psychological health, and this app-roach has been previously applied for other injuries and disorders, such as brachial plexus birth injury [18] as well as orofacial cleft [19]. In the unadjusted analysis, both absolute and relative risk of psychotropic medication use was much higher in individuals that were diagnosed and surgically treated for CTS and UNE or both conditions. The combination of these two nerve compression disorders simultaneously is not common from a population perspective, but rather common from a clinical perspective as to why the individuals appearing with such a combination were also included in the present study [2]. In the regression models, we found that this increased risk of psychotropic drug use in surgically treated individuals with CTS, UNE and the combination of CTS and UNE remained when adjusted for age, sex, income, country of birth and occupational qualifications with PRs of about 1.50. In the same models, PRs for the use of psychotropic drugs were also increased by a higher age, being a woman, having low income and a low occupational qualification level. Regarding the relevance of these factors, one may consider that socioeconomic status can be a confounder from the perspective of nerve compression disorders and impaired psychological health. However, our adjusted analyses (Table 2, model 2) indicated an independent effect of both the nerve compression disorders and the socioeconomic status. A positive association between anxiety, depression, and health-related quality of life with patient-reported symptom severity, but not for objectively derived severity, of CTS has been reported [25]. Some authors argue that electrophysiological testing, as a more objective assessment, should be performed before considering surgery in CTS due to the risk that poor mental health results in functional symptoms [26].

There are socioeconomic disparities among individuals surgically treated for CTS, where socially deprived patients are less likely to receive surgical treatment in an American setting [11]. Whether this is also the case in countries such as Sweden, where health care is financed by the government and equally available regardless of socioeconomic status, remains unknown. However, in our database most patients with a diagnosis received surgical treatment. Economic well-being seems to be crucial in CTS since a low economic well-being is related to higher comorbidity burden [12], such as diabetes in which nerves are more susceptible to nerve compression [27,28]. There is also evidence that both type of occupation as well as level of educational achievement are important for development of clinically relevant CTS [7]. Most of these socioeconomical factors are associated with more symptoms both before and after surgery for CTS, but do not affect the relative improvement [9]. Analysis of preoperative psychological mindsets, based on several questionnaires, seems to be important for predicting the outcome of surgery [29]. Return to work after surgery for CTS is also influenced by illness perception and mental health [17], which seems to be particularly relevant for treated women for CTS where depression predicts outcome [16]. In the present study, a low income as well as a low occupational qualification level were associated with an increased odds ratio for use of psychotropic drugs over and above other factors. Thus, the etiological factors, often multifactorial, behind nerve compression disorders, such as CTS and the relation to mental health, such as depression and socioeconomic status, are complex, but should be considered in clinical practice when treating individuals with nerve compression disorders.

Most studies concerning the importance of mental illness and socioeconomical factors for having or being treated for a nerve compression disorder have so far been focused on CTS and there have been few on UNE [13]. CTS and UNE, requiring surgery, are more common in socially deprived individuals and seem to occur at an earlier age [15], where the authors stressed that the relationship was strikingly similar for UNE and CTS. We found a higher risk for use of psychotropic drugs among the surgically treated individuals with CTS, UNE and the combination of UNE and CTS, although the size of the risk was different between the three groups. The high use of psychotropic drugs among middle aged women with UNE is an interesting observation. Despite some similarities between CTS and UNE as nerve compression disorders, the latter condition is different in many aspects. This includes a more unpredictable outcome of surgery in some individuals with UNE, where psychological health may be one crucial influencing factor and a risk for postoperative neuropathic pain. Thus, the indication for surgery for UNE should be very clear and sometimes strict. An interesting question is if patients with preoperative anxiety and/or depression benefit from a specific type of surgery, but data indicate that patients, surgically treated with a total knee arthroplasty, are improved regardless of their presurgical psychological status [30]. Preoperative information, where also assessment of the psychological and psychiatric status is considered before surgery, seems to be crucial [31] and anxiety and depression symptoms may also decrease after a total knee arthroplasty [32]. Finally, we did not find any positive association between country of birth and the diagnosis or treatment of the three disorders; in fact, model 2 of the regression analysis indicated a decreased use of psychotropic drugs in surgically treated individuals born outside of Sweden. However, it is known that there is an underutilization of health care services and especially psychiatric medication by migrants [33,34].

Our study has several strengths. It is based on large national registers that cover the whole Swedish population and all the relevant patients. The coding of the diagnoses and surgical procedures is also highly standardized and similar across the whole country. However, it might also have some limitations. For instance, one may argue that our study did not have data from primary health care, but we defined the exposed population as patients diagnosed and surgically treated for a nerve compression disorder, which is a clear and valid definition of such syndromes, excluding transient and possibly vague symptoms from the peripheral nervous system. We also excluded 423,414 individuals residing less than five years in Sweden. We did so because it is known that there is an underutilization of health care services by migrants, especially those residing for only a few years in the country [34]. In addition, we aimed to obtain a solid measure of socioeconomic position based on information about income during the last 10 years and to obtain information about previous use of psychotropic medication and relevant surgery.

We conclude, based on a large record linkage database of several national registers covering the entire Swedish population at the age of 25–<80 years, that surgically treated individuals suffering from a nerve compression disorder, such as CTS and particularly UNE and a combination of both disorders, have an increased risk of impaired psychological health as expressed by their high use of psychotropic medication, and this risk is independent of the socioeconomic characteristics of the patients. Caregivers involved in the treatment of individuals with nerve compression disorders should be aware of such an increased risk and be ready to provide the necessary attention to the individual.

Author Contributions: Conceptualization, L.B.D., E.N., M.Z. and J.M.; Methodology, L.B.D., R.P. and J.M.; Software, R.P. and J.M. Validation, R.P.; Formal Analysis, R.P. and J.M.; Investigation, L.B.D., E.N., M.Z., R.P. and J.M.; Resources, L.B.D., E.N., M.Z. and J.M. Data Curation, R.P. and J.M.; Writing original draft, L.B.D., E.N., M.Z., R.P. and J.M. All authors have read and agreed to the published version of the manuscript.

Funding: This research was funded by the Swedish Research Council (# 2017-01321. Principal investigator: JM; #2022-01942, principal investigator LBD), the Swedish Diabetes Foundation (#DIA2020-492), the Regional Agreement on Medical Training and Clinical Research (ALF; PI Dahlin) between Region Skåne and Lund University (#2018-Projekt0104; PI Dahlin) and Funds from Skåne University Hospital (#2019-659; PI Dahlin), Elly Olsson´s Foundation for scientific research, Stig and Ragna Gorthon Foundation, Almroth Foundation, Kockska foundation, the Magnus Bergvall Foundation [2020-03612].

Institutional Review Board Statement: The record linkage was performed using a unique personal identification number and it was facilitated by the National Board of Health and Welfare and Statistics Sweden after revision and consent by their own data safety committees and initial approval by the Regional Ethical Committee in South Sweden (#: 2014-856). The Swedish authorities anonymized the database before delivering it to us.

Informed Consent Statement: Patient consent was waived due to the data consisted of data obtained from national registers in Sweden with anonymized data as approved by the National Ethical Committee.

Data Availability Statement: Relevant data are included within the paper. The complete and detailed individual data of all subjects cannot be publicly available for ethical and/or legal reasons due to compromising patient privacy. The Regional and National Ethical Committee have imposed these restrictions. Data requests may be sent to The National Ethical Committee via the homepage of Etikprövningsmyndigheten in Sweden (etikprovningsmyndigheten.se, accessed on 1 June 2022). The database we analyzed is not publicly available for ethical and data safety reasons. However, the same dataset can be constructed by request to the Swedish National Board of Health and Welfare and Statistics Sweden after approval of the research project by an Ethical Committee and by the data safety committees of the Swedish Authorities. The study also needs to be performed in collaboration with Swedish researchers. [1] 1. Public Access to Information Secrecy Act. In: Justice Mo, editor. Stockholm2009.

Acknowledgments: The authors would like to thank Tina Folker for her administrative support.

Conflicts of Interest: The authors declare no conflict of interest. The funders had no role in the design of the study; in the collection, analyses, or interpretation of data; in the writing of the manuscript, or in the decision to publish the results.

References

1. Bartels, R.H.; Verbeek, A.L. Risk factors for ulnar nerve compression at the elbow: A case control study. *Acta Neurochir.* **2007**, *149*, 669–674; discussion 674. [CrossRef] [PubMed]
2. Giostad, A.; Nyman, E. Patient Characteristics in Ulnar Nerve Compression at the Elbow at a Tertiary Referral Hospital and Predictive Factors for Outcomes of Simple Decompression versus Subcutaneous Transposition of the Ulnar Nerve. *Biomed. Res. Int.* **2019**, *2019*, 5302462. [CrossRef] [PubMed]
3. Anker, I.; Zimmerman, M.; Andersson, G.S.; Jacobsson, H.; Dahlin, L.B. Outcome and predictors in simple decompression of ulnar nerve entrapment at the elbow. *Hand Microsurg.* **2018**, *7*, 24–32. [CrossRef]
4. Giostad, A.; Rantfors, R.; Nyman, T.; Nyman, E. Enrollment in Treatment at a Specialized Pain Management Clinic at a Tertiary Referral Center after Surgery for Ulnar Nerve Compression: Patient Characteristics and Outcome. *J. Hand Surg. Glob. Online* **2021**, *3*, 110–116. [CrossRef] [PubMed]
5. Hulkkonen, S.; Lampainen, K.; Auvinen, J.; Miettunen, J.; Karppinen, J.; Ryhänen, J. Incidence and operations of median, ulnar and radial entrapment neuropathies in Finland: A nationwide register study. *J. Hand Surg.* **2020**, *45*, 226–230. [CrossRef]
6. Pourmemari, M.H.; Heliovaara, M.; Viikari-Juntura, E.; Shiri, R. Carpal tunnel release: Lifetime prevalence, annual incidence, and risk factors. *Muscle Nerve* **2018**, *58*, 497–502. [CrossRef]
7. Mollestam, K.; Englund, M.; Atroshi, I. Association of clinically relevant carpal tunnel syndrome with type of work and level of education: A general-population study. *Sci. Rep.* **2021**, *11*, 19850. [CrossRef]
8. Jenkins, P.J.; Watts, A.C.; Duckworth, A.D.; McEachan, J.E. Socioeconomic deprivation and the epidemiology of carpal tunnel syndrome. *J. Hand Surg.* **2012**, *37E*, 123–129. [CrossRef]
9. Zimmerman, M.; Hall, E.; Carlsson, K.S.; Nyman, E.; Dahlin, L.B. Socioeconomic factors predicting outcome in surgically treated carpal tunnel syndrome: A national registry-based study. *Sci. Rep.* **2021**, *11*, 2581. [CrossRef]
10. Goodson, J.T.; DeBerard, M.S.; Wheeler, A.J.; Colledge, A.L. Occupational and biopsychosocial risk factors for carpal tunnel syndrome. *J. Occup. Environ. Med.* **2014**, *56*, 965–972. [CrossRef]
11. Brodeur, P.G.; Patel, D.D.; Licht, A.H.; Loftus, D.H.; Cruz, A.I., Jr.; Gil, J.A. Demographic Disparities amongst Patients Receiving Carpal Tunnel Release: A Retrospective Review of 92,921 Patients. *Plast. Reconstr. Surg. Glob. Open* **2021**, *9*, e3959. [CrossRef] [PubMed]
12. Zhang, D.; Earp, B.E.; Blazar, P. Association of Economic Well-Being with Comorbid Conditions in Patients Undergoing Carpal Tunnel Release. *J. Hand Surg. Am.* **2021**. [CrossRef]
13. Zimmerman, M.; Nyman, E.; Steen Carlsson, K.; Dahlin, L.B. Socioeconomic Factors in Patients with Ulnar Nerve Compression at the Elbow: A National Registry-Based Study. *Biomed. Res. Int.* **2020**, *2020*, 5928469. [CrossRef] [PubMed]
14. Hulkkonen, S.; Auvinen, J.; Miettunen, J.; Karppinen, J.; Ryhanen, J. Smoking is associated with ulnar nerve entrapment: A birth cohort study. *Sci. Rep.* **2019**, *9*, 9450. [CrossRef] [PubMed]

15. Johnson, N.A.; Darwin, O.; Chasiouras, D.; Selby, A.; Bainbridge, C. The effect of social deprivation on the incidence rate of carpal and cubital tunnel syndrome surgery. *J. Hand Surg.* **2021**, *46*, 265–269. [CrossRef]
16. Fernandez-de-Las-Penas, C.; de-la-Llave-Rincon, A.I.; Cescon, C.; Barbero, M.; Arias-Buria, J.L.; Falla, D. Influence of Clinical, Psychological, and Psychophysical Variables on Long-term Treatment Outcomes in Carpal Tunnel Syndrome: Evidence from a Randomized Clinical Trial. *Pain Pract.* **2019**, *19*, 644–655. [CrossRef] [PubMed]
17. Jansen, M.C.; van der Oest, M.J.W.; de Haas, N.P.; Selles Ph, D.R.; Zuidam Md Ph, D.J.; Hand-Wrist Study, G. The Influence of Illness Perception and Mental Health on Return to Work After Carpal Tunnel Release Surgery. *J. Hand Surg. Am.* **2021**, *46*, 748–757. [CrossRef]
18. Psouni, E.; Perez Vicente, R.; Dahlin, L.B.; Merlo, J. Psychotropic drug use as indicator of mental health in adolescents affected by a plexus injury at birth: A large population-based study in Sweden. *PLoS ONE* **2018**, *13*, e0193635. [CrossRef]
19. Nilsson, S.; Merlo, J.; Lyberg-Ahlander, V.; Psouni, E. Psychotropic drug use in adolescents born with an orofacial cleft: A population-based study. *BMJ Open* **2015**, *5*, e005306. [CrossRef]
20. Johnson, N.A.; Darwin, O.; Chasiouras, D.; Selby, A.; Bainbridge, C. The association between surgery for carpal and cubital tunnel syndrome: Analysis of incidence and risk factors within a geographical area. *J. Hand Surg.* **2021**, *46*, 260–264. [CrossRef]
21. Statistics Sweden. MIS 2012:1, SSYK 2012 Swedish Standard Classification of Occupations 2012. Available online: https://www.scb.se/contentassets/c9d055b6f2114b62bd23c33602b56da5/ov9999_2012a01_br_x70br1201.pdf (accessed on 1 January 2022).
22. Barros, A.J.; Hirakata, V.N. Alternatives for logistic regression in cross-sectional studies: An empirical comparison of models that directly estimate the prevalence ratio. *BMC Med. Res. Methodol.* **2003**, *3*, 21. [CrossRef] [PubMed]
23. Pepe, M.S.; Janes, H.; Longton, G.; Leisenring, W.; Newcomb, P. Limitations of the odds ratio in gauging the performance of a diagnostic, prognostic, or screening marker. *Am. J. Epidemiol.* **2004**, *159*, 882–890. [CrossRef] [PubMed]
24. Hosmer, D.W.; Lemeshow, S. *Applied Logistic Regression*, 2nd ed.; Wiley: New York, NY, USA, 2000.
25. Jerosch-Herold, C.; Houghton, J.; Blake, J.; Shaikh, A.; Wilson, E.C.; Shepstone, L. Association of psychological distress, quality of life and costs with carpal tunnel syndrome severity: A cross-sectional analysis of the PALMS cohort. *BMJ Open* **2017**, *7*, e017732. [CrossRef] [PubMed]
26. McCallum, L.M.; Damms, N.A.; Sarrigiannis, P.G.; Zis, P. Anxiety and depression in patients with suspected carpal tunnel syndrome—A case-controlled study. *Brain Behav.* **2019**, *9*, e01342. [CrossRef]
27. Zimmerman, M.; Gottsäter, A.; Dahlin, L.B. Carpal Tunnel Syndrome and Diabetes-A Comprehensive Review. *J. Clin. Med.* **2022**, *11*, 1674. [CrossRef]
28. Rydberg, M.; Zimmerman, M.; Gottsater, A.; Nilsson, P.M.; Melander, O.; Dahlin, L.B. Diabetes mellitus as a risk factor for compression neuropathy: A longitudinal cohort study from southern Sweden. *BMJ Open Diabetes Res. Care* **2020**, *8*, e001298. [CrossRef]
29. Sun, P.O.; Walbeehm, E.T.; Selles, R.W.; Slijper, H.P.; Ulrich, D.J.O.; Porsius, J.T.; Hand Wrist Study, G. Patient Mindset and the Success of Carpal Tunnel Release. *Plast. Reconstr. Surg.* **2021**, *147*, 66e–75e. [CrossRef]
30. Mahdi, A.; Halleberg-Nyman, M.; Wretenberg, P. Preoperative psychological distress no reason to delay total knee arthroplasty: A register-based prospective cohort study of 458 patients. *Arch. Orthop. Trauma Surg.* **2020**, *140*, 1809–1818. [CrossRef]
31. Mahdi, A.; Nyman, M.H.; Wretenberg, P. How do orthopaedic surgeons inform their patients before knee arthroplasty surgery? A cross-sectional study. *BMC Musculoskelet. Disord.* **2018**, *19*, 414. [CrossRef]
32. Mahdi, A. Psychological Distress and Contentment after Primary Total Knee Replacement. Ph.D. Thesis, Örebro University, Örebro, Sweden, 2020.
33. Moradi, F. No integration without health. *Lakartidningen* **2013**, *110*, 1046.
34. Graetz, V.; Rechel, B.; Groot, W.; Norredam, M.; Pavlova, M. Utilization of health care services by migrants in Europe-a systematic literature review. *Br. Med. Bull.* **2017**, *121*, 5–18. [CrossRef] [PubMed]

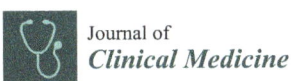

Article

Electrodiagnostic Testing and Nerve Ultrasound of the Carpal Tunnel in Patients with Type 2 Diabetes

Bianka Heiling [1,2,*], Leonie I. E. E. Wiedfeld [1], Nicolle Müller [3], Niklas J. Kobler [1], Alexander Grimm [4], Christof Kloos [3] and Hubertus Axer [1]

1. Department of Neurology, Jena University Hospital, Friedrich Schiller University, 07747 Jena, Germany; leonie.wiedfeld@med.uni-jena.de (L.I.E.E.W.); niklasjohannes.kobler@med.uni-jena.de (N.J.K.); hubertus.axer@med.uni-jena.de (H.A.)
2. Clinician Scientist Program OrganAge, Jena University Hospital, 07747 Jena, Germany
3. Department of Internal Medicine III, Jena University Hospital, Friedrich Schiller University, 07747 Jena, Germany; nicolle.mueller@med.uni-jena.de (N.M.); christof.kloos@med.uni-jena.de (C.K.)
4. Department of Neurology, Tuebingen University Hospital, 72076 Tuebingen, Germany; alexander.grimm@med.uni-tuebingen.de
* Correspondence: bianka.heiling@med.uni-jena.de

Abstract: In diabetic patients, controversies still exist about the validity of electrodiagnostic and nerve ultrasound diagnosis for carpal tunnel syndrome (CTS). We analyzed 69 patients with type 2 diabetes. Nerve conduction studies and peripheral nerve ultrasound of the median nerve over the carpal tunnel were performed. CTS symptoms were assessed using the Boston Carpal Tunnel Questionnaire. Polyneuropathy was assessed using the Neuropathy Symptom Score and the Neuropathy Disability Score. Although 19 patients reported predominantly mild CTS symptoms, 37 patients met the electrophysiological diagnosis criteria for CTS, and six patients were classified as severe or extremely severe. The sonographic cross-sectional area (CSA) of the median nerve at the wrist was larger than 12 mm^2 in 45 patients (65.2%), and the wrist-to-forearm-ratio was larger than 1.4 in 61 patients (88.4%). Receiver operating characteristic analysis showed that neither the distal motor latency, the median nerve CSA, nor the wrist-to-forearm-ratio could distinguish between patients with and without CTS symptoms. Diagnosis of CTS in diabetic patients should primarily be based upon typical clinical symptoms and signs. Results of electrodiagnostic testing and nerve ultrasound have to be interpreted with caution and additional factors have to be considered especially polyneuropathy, but also body mass index and hyperglycemia.

Keywords: carpal tunnel syndrome; diabetes mellitus; nerve conduction study; peripheral nerve ultrasound

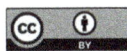

1. Introduction

Carpal tunnel syndrome (CTS) is the most common entrapment neuropathy in the general population [1]. Risk factors for CTS are diabetes mellitus, obesity, metabolic syndrome, thyroid dysfunction, rheumatic diseases, and others [2,3]. It has been shown that the incidence of CTS is increased in diabetic patients [4]. Typical symptoms are numbness, predominantly nocturnal par- and dysesthesias, and/or neuropathic pain, which are associated with localized compression of the median nerve at the wrist, and weakness and atrophy of the thenar muscle later in the course of the disease [5,6].

Nerve conduction studies are the technical gold standard for diagnosis [7]. CTS typically shows an elongation of the distal motor latency (DML) and a decrease in sensory nerve conduction velocity (CV) measured over the wrist. Principally, sensory changes occur before motor changes and changes in latencies and CV precedes changes in the amplitudes of compound motor action potentials (CMAP) and sensory nerve action potentials (SNAP). It is recommended that nerve conduction studies for the diagnosis of CTS be performed in patients with clinical manifestations of CTS [8].

Recently, peripheral nerve ultrasound was revealed to give valuable additional information; so, it has been advised to perform nerve ultrasound in addition to electrodiagnostic testing [9]. Sonographic diagnosis is based on a swelling of the median nerve at the inlet of the carpal tunnel (at the level of the pisiform bone), where an increase in the cross-sectional area (CSA) of the median nerve can be measured [10,11]. In addition, the wrist-to-forearm-ratio (WFR) compares the median nerve CSA at the wrist to the CSA 12 cm proximal at the forearm and shows a high sensitivity to detect CTS if the ratio is larger than 1.4 [12].

However, in diabetic patients, still controversies and uncertainties exist as to how far the diagnosis criteria for CTS may be valid for electrodiagnostic testing [13,14] and nerve ultrasound as well [15]. A major factor is generally seen in the coexistence of diabetic neuropathy, which also influences carpal tunnel measurements [16]. Most of the studies evaluated diabetic patients with the clinical diagnosis of CTS.

The clinical question here is how to interpret electrodiagnostic testing and ultrasound results for suspected CTS in patients with type 2 diabetes. Therefore, the aim of this study is to analyze patients with type 2 diabetes independent from the medical history of CTS or diabetic neuropathy in order to compare CTS symptoms (measured by the Boston Carpal Tunnel Questionnaire), diabetic neuropathy, nerve conduction studies, and peripheral nerve ultrasound of the median nerve.

2. Materials and Methods

2.1. Patients

We analyzed a database of patients with type 2 diabetes mellitus who participated in the still-ongoing SELECT study (Sonographic and electrophysiological characterization of peripheral nerves in patients with type 2 diabetes, German Clinical Trials Register DRKS00023026). All patients presented in the tertiary care outpatient clinic for diabetology at Jena University Hospital. The data were collected prospectively between September 2020 and April 2022. All participants gave written informed consent. The study was approved by the local ethics committee (number 2019-1416-BO).

Inclusion criteria were patients with type 2 diabetes, age between 40 and 85 years, willing to fill out questionnaires, and willing to undergo nerve conduction studies and peripheral nerve ultrasound. Exclusion criteria were known other etiologies for polyneuropathy (such as alcohol abuse, inflammatory polyneuropathies, etc.), rheumatic disease, peripheral arterial occlusive disease, active malignant tumor disease, and history of chemotherapy and CTS surgery.

2.2. Assessments

Several baseline parameters were collected: age, gender, duration of diabetes in years, body mass index (kg/m^2), HbA$_{1c}$ (mmol/mol), and glomerular filtration rate (mL/min). HbA$_{1c}$ was measured using high-performance liquid chromatography (TOSOH-Glykohaemoglobin-Analyzer HLC-723 GhbV, Tosoh Corporation, Tokyo, Japan).

Symptoms and deficits due to CTS were inquired using the Boston Carpal Tunnel Questionnaire (BCTQ) [17], which consisted of two parts: the Symptom Severity Scale (SSS) and the Functional Status Scale (FSS). The SSS included eleven questions and the answers ranged from 1 (no pain or difficulties) to 5 (severe/permanent pain or difficulties). The score (ranging from 11 to 55) discerns five degrees of severity (0 = asymptomatic to 4 = severely affected). The SSS is performed for each hand separately. The FSS includes eight activities in daily life, which are scored from 1 (no difficulties) to 5 (not feasible). The score (ranging from 8 to 40) also discerns five degrees of severity (0 = asymptomatic to 4 = severely affected). The German version of the BCTQ has been shown to have sufficient internal consistency, reliability, and validity to assess the health status in CTS [18].

Subjective symptoms due to diabetic polyneuropathy were evaluated using the Neuropathy Symptom Score (NSS) and the severity of sensory deficits using the Neuropathy Disability Score (NDS) [19]. NSS asks for sensory symptoms in the legs (burning, numbness, tingling, fatigue, cramping), the localization, time of appearance, and improvements.

Scores of 3–4 imply mild, 5–6 moderate, and 7–10 severe symptoms. The NDS checks ankle reflexes, vibration perception threshold (tuning fork), pain sensitivity (pin-prick), and temperature sensitivity. Scores of 3–5 imply mild, 6–8 moderate, and 9–10 severe deficits. Based on NSS and NDS scores, diabetic polyneuropathy can be diagnosed; if the NDS is between 6 and 8 or NDS is between 3 and 5 and NSS is between 5 and 6 [20].

Principally, the right median nerve was measured with nerve conduction studies (NCS) and peripheral nerve ultrasound, except if there was a pathology at the right wrist (such as complex regional pain syndrome, amputation, status after surgery, fractures, and others). In this exception, the left median nerve was measured (in 11 patients). The examiner was blinded with respect to the existence of CTS symptoms.

Nerve conduction studies (NCS) of the median nerve were performed by an experienced neurologist using a Medelec Synergy device (Synergy 15.0; Viasys Healthcare, Natus Europe GmbH, Planegg, Germany). Measurements were carried out on the median nerve (on the same side as the ultrasound measurements). Here, we measured the distal motor latency (DML), the amplitude of compound muscle action potential (CMAP) of the abductor pollicis brevis muscle, the sensory nerve conduction velocity (CV), and the amplitude of the sensory nerve action potential (SNAP) measured at the second finger (Figure 1A–C). The distance over the wrist between stimulation and recording electrode for motor NCS was kept constant at 7 to 8 cm. Skin temperature was controlled to be between 32 and 34 °C. Cut-off values in our laboratory for the median nerve are (according to [21]) DML 4.2 ms, CMAP amplitude 5.0 mV, sensory CV 45 m/s, and SNAP amplitude 6.9 µV.

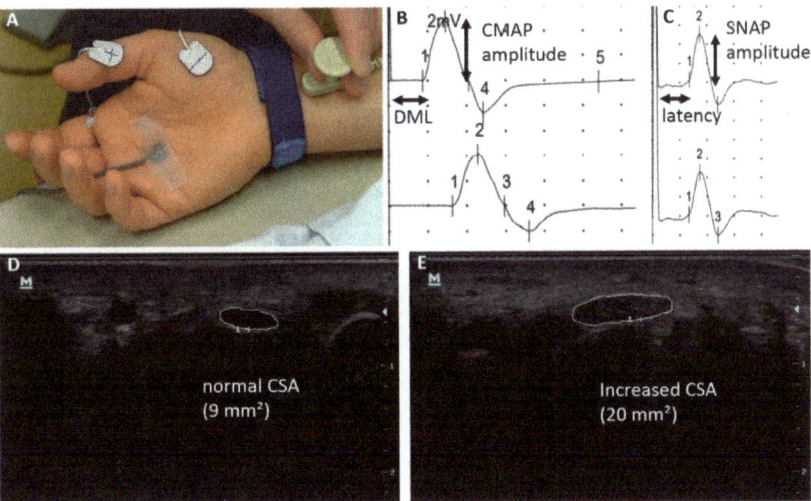

Figure 1. Nerve conduction studies and peripheral nerve ultrasound of the median nerve at the wrist. (**A**) Placement of electrodes. (**B**) Motor nerve conduction study. (**C**) Sensory nerve conduction study. (**D**) Normal cross-sectional area (CSA) of the median nerve. (**E**) Increased CSA of the median nerve. Abbreviations: CMAP, compound motor action potential; CSA, cross-sectional area; DML, distal motor latency; SNAP, sensory nerve action potential.

Sonographic examinations were performed by an experienced neurologist using a high-resolution ultrasound device (Mindray M7, Medical Australia Ltd., Ultrasound systems, Darmstadt, Germany) with a 14 MHz linear-array transducer. The median nerve was measured at the inlet of the carpal tunnel (at the level of the pisiform bone) and 12 cm proximal of the wrist at the forearm. We measured the CSA using direct-tracing technique around the inner margin of the hyperechoic epineural sheath (Figure 1B,D) and calculated the wrist-to-forearm-ratio. For the CSA of the median nerve at the level of the pisiforme bone, a cut-off value of 10 mm^2 showed good diagnostic utility and a wrist-to-forearm-ratio of ≥ 1.4 showed a high sensitivity in the general population [22].

2.3. Statistics

All data were analyzed with the Statistical Package for the Social Sciences software (SPSS version 25.0; IBM Corporation, Armonk, NY, USA). The values were presented as mean and standard deviation (SD) or as numbers and percentages. First, we described the cohort using descriptive statistics.

Spearman correlations were used to analyze correlations between nerve conduction studies and peripheral nerve ultrasound. Unpaired t-test was used to analyze differences of measurements between patients with and without CTS symptoms and between patients with and without diabetic polyneuropathy. Linear regression was used to evaluate potential influences of clinical parameters on electrodiagnostic measurements and sonographic measurements. Finally, receiver operating characteristic (ROC) analysis was used to evaluate the potential of these measurements to differentiate between patients with and without CTS symptoms. For all analyses, a p value < 0.05 was considered statistically significant.

3. Results

3.1. Patients

At the time point of analysis, 88 patients were included in the SELECT cohort and were screened for eligibility for this study. Nine patients had CTS surgery before and 10 patients did not answer the BCTQ. Therefore, 19 patients had to be excluded from analysis. Thus, 69 patients with type 2 diabetes (26 female and 43 male) were finally included into this study. Tables 1 and 2 show the baseline characteristics of the patients. Fifty patients reported no CTS typical symptoms at the analyzed hand (BCTQ SSS = 0) and 19 patients only reported predominantly mild CTS symptoms. In contrast, 49 patients were diagnosed having typical signs of diabetic polyneuropathy (when NDS was between 6 and 8 or NDS was between 3 and 5 and NSS was between 5 and 6, according to [20]).

Table 1. Baseline characteristics of the patients (n = 69), categorical variables.

Variable		n	%
Sex	Female	26	37.7
	Male	43	62.3
BCTQ SSS at the measured hand	0	50	72.5
	1	17	24.6
	2	1	1.4
	3	1	1.4
BCTQ SSS right hand	0	50	72.5
	1	17	24.6
	2	1	1.4
	3	1	1.4
BCTQ SSS left hand	0	51	73.9
	1	16	23.2
	2	1	1.4
	3	1	1.4
BCTQ FSS	0	50	72.5
	1	18	26.1
	4	1	1.4
Polyneuropathy if NDS > 5 or (NDS > 2 and NSS > 4)	Yes	49	71.0
	No	20	29.0

Table 1. Cont.

Variable		n	%
NSS	No symptoms (0–2)	27	39.1
	Mild symptoms (3–4)	10	14.5
	Moderate symptoms (5–6)	16	23.2
	Severe symptoms (7–10)	17	24.6
NDS	No deficits (0–2)	9	13.2
	Mild deficits (3–5)	18	26.5
	Moderate deficits (6–8)	26	38.2
	Severe deficits (9–10)	15	22.1
CTS symptoms and diabetic polyneuropathy	Asymptomatic + no neuropathy	18	26.1
	CTS symptoms only	2	0.3
	Diabetic neuropathy only	32	46.4
	CTS symptoms and neuropathy	17	24.6

Abbreviations: BCTQ, Boston Carpal Tunnel Questionnaire; FSS, Functional Status Scale; NDS, Neuropathy Disability Score; NSS, Neuropathy Symptom Score; SSS, Symptom Severity Scale.

Table 2. Baseline characteristics of the patients (n = 69), metric variables.

Variable	Mean	SD	Minimum	Maximum
Age (years)	66.77	9.72	44	82
Duration of diabetes (years)	14.72	8.95	0.63	38
Body mass index (kg/m^2)	32.42	6.17	20.1	48.0
HbA$_{1c}$ (mmol/mol)	59.08	10.94	27.98	82.51
Glomerular filtration rate (mL/min)	71.79	20.64	27.92	107.25
CSA median nerve at wrist (mm^2)	13.53	4.74	5.00	37.00
CSA median nerve at forearm (mm^2)	7.03	2.09	4.00	15.00
Wrist-to-forearm-ratio	2.05	0.76	0.33	4.75
Distal motor latency median nerve (ms)	4.42	0.67	3.50	6.15
CMAP amplitude median nerve (mV)	10.12	4.39	0	22.30
Sensory nerve CV median nerve (m/s)	43.26	7.84	29.0	63.6
SNAP amplitude median nerve (µV)	13.31	9.64	0	48.9
NSS (0–10 points)	3.84	3.23	0	9
NDS (0–10 points)	6.10	2.75	0	10

Abbreviations: CMAP, compound motor action potential; CSA, cross-sectional area; CV, conduction velocity; NDS, Neuropathy Disability Score; NSS, Neuropathy Symptom Score; SNAP, sensory nerve action potential.

3.2. Nerve Conduction Studies

Distal motor latencies of the right median nerve larger than 4.2 ms were found in 34 patients, and in two patients, no CMAP could be measured. Thirty-four patients showed sensory nerve conduction velocities slower than 45 m/s and five patients had no SNAPs. Figure 2 shows the measurements of nerve conduction studies. As expected, there was a correlation between DML and sensory conduction velocity (Spearman correlation coefficient of −0.532, $p < 0.001$). Using the Bland classification of neurophysiological severity of CTS [23], nine patients showed mild, twenty-two moderate, four severe, and two extremely severe neurophysiological measurements.

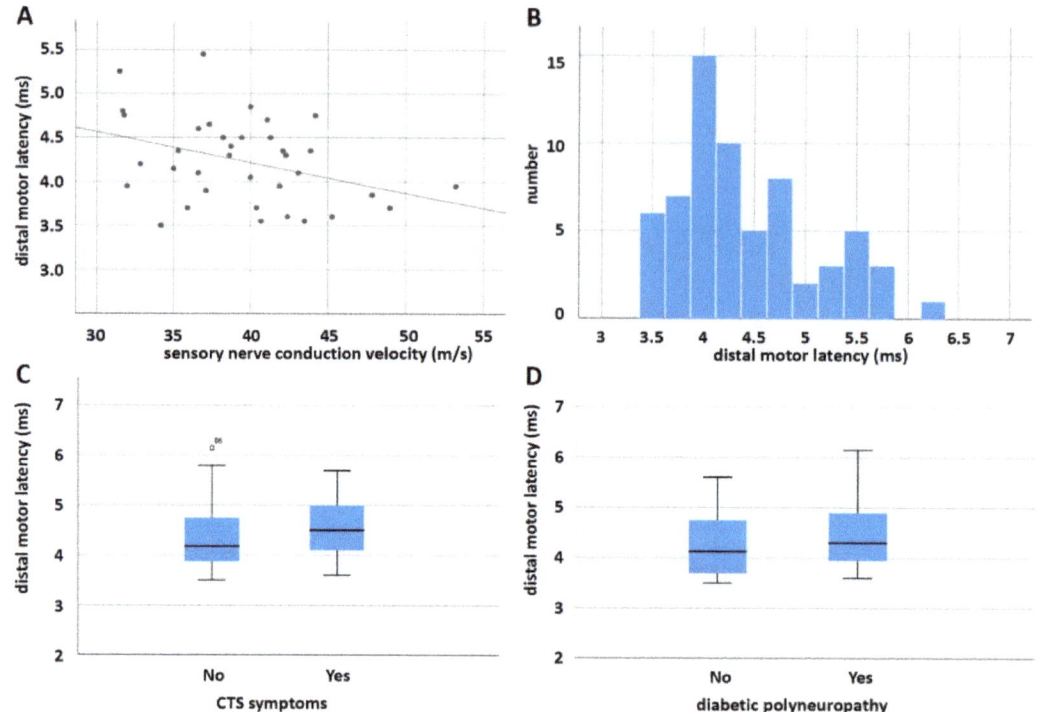

Figure 2. Nerve conduction studies of the median nerve. (**A**) Scatter plot of sensory nerve conduction velocity and distal motor latency. (**B**) Histogram of distal motor latencies. (**C**) Box plots of distal motor latencies in patients with and without CTS symptoms. (**D**) Box plots of distal motor latencies in patients with and without diabetic polyneuropathy.

DML did not show statistically significant differences between patients with and without CTS symptoms (Figure 2C, t-test: T = 1.151, p = 0.254) and between patients with and without diabetic polyneuropathy (Figure 2D, t-test: T = 1.465, p = 0.148).

3.3. Peripheral Nerve Ultrasound

Median nerve CSA at the wrist was between 10 and 12 mm^2 in 16 patients, between 12 and 15 mm^2 in 24 patients, and larger than 15 mm^2 in 21 patients. Sixty-one patients had a WFR $\geq$ 1.4. Figure 3 shows the ultrasound measurements of the median nerve.

Median nerve CSA at the wrist and wrist-to-forearm-ratio did not show any statistically significant differences between patients with and without CTS symptoms (Figure 3C, CSA: t-test, T = 0.621, p = 0.537; wrist-to-forearm-ratio: t-test, T = 0.161, p = 0.873) nor between patients with and without diabetic polyneuropathy (Figure 3D, CSA: t-test, T = 1.273, p = 0.207; wrist-to-forearm-ratio: t-test, T = 0.120, p = 0.905).

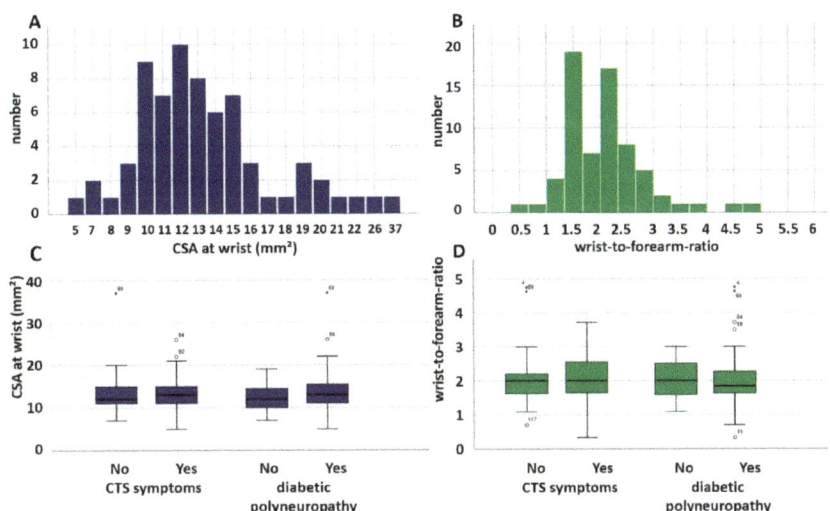

Figure 3. Peripheral nerve ultrasound measurements of the median nerve at the wrist. (**A**) Histogram of the CSA at the wrist. (**B**) Histogram of the wrist-to-forearm-ratio. (**C**) Box plots of median nerve CSA at the wrist in patients with and without CTS symptoms and patients with and without diabetic polyneuropathy. (**D**) Box plots of wrist-to-forearm-ratio in patients with and without CTS symptoms and patients with and without diabetic polyneuropathy.

3.4. Interactions

A correlation (Figure 4) between DML and median nerve CSA at the wrist (Spearman correlation coefficient of 0.406, $p = 0.001$) and between DML and wrist-to-forearm-ratio (Spearman correlation coefficient of 0.324, $p = 0.009$) could be found.

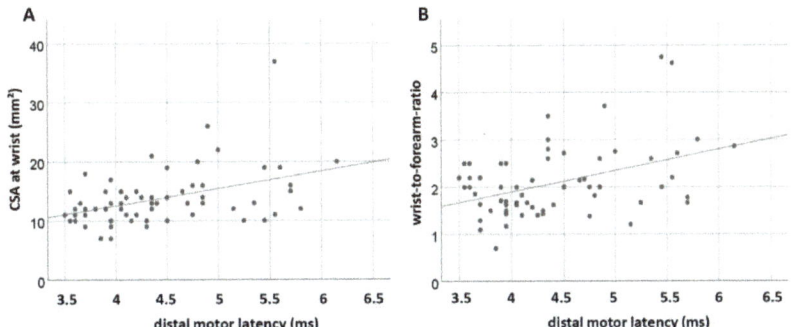

Figure 4. Scatterplots of distal motor latencies and peripheral nerve ultrasound measurements. (**A**) Distal motor latencies and median nerve CSA at the wrist. (**B**) Distal motor latencies and wrist-to-forearm-ratio.

Linear regression showed body mass index being a predictive variable for median nerve CSA and HbA_{1c} being a predictive variable for wrist-to-forearm-ratio (Table 3), although both had small R^2 (0.065 and 0.068, respectively).

Table 3. Linear regression.

Variable	Coefficient	Standard Error	p	Beta
Model1 with median nerve CSA as dependent variable ($R^2 = 0.065$)				
Constant	7.269	8.375	0.027	
Body mass index	0.197	0.102	0.047	0.255
Model2 with wrist-to-forearm-ration as dependent variable ($R^2 = 0.068$)				
Constant	1.036	3.206	0.052	
HbA_{1c}	0.018	0.097	0.043	0.260

Receiver operating characteristic (ROC) analysis showed that neither distal motor latency, cross-sectional area of the median nerve at the wrist, nor the wrist-to-forearm-ratio were able to distinguish between diabetic patients with and without symptoms for CTS (Figure 5). Area under the curve was 0.632 for the distal motor latency, 0.473 for the median nerve CSA, and 0.546 for the wrist-to-forearm-ratio.

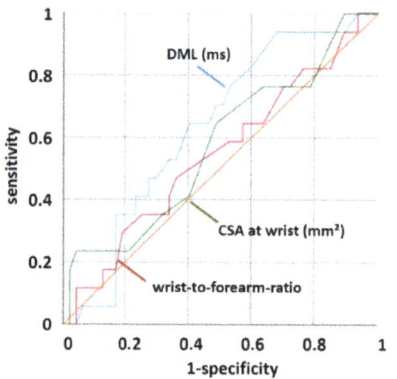

Figure 5. ROC curve analysis shows that DML, median nerve CSA at the wrist, and wrist-to-forearm-ratio were not suited to distinguish between diabetic patients with and without symptoms for CTS.

4. Discussion

Symptoms characteristic of CTS such as pain, numbness, and/or tingling in the median nerve distribution in the hands have been shown to have a prevalence of 14.4% in the general population, while CTS typical changes in nerve conduction studies of the median nerve have a prevalence of 4.9% [24]. According to the clinical diagnosis of CTS, the prevalence of CTS was 2% in the general population, 14% in diabetic patients without neuropathy, and 30% in patients with diabetic neuropathy [13].

In our study, patients with type 2 diabetes were examined regardless of having CTS or not. In this cohort, 50 patients did not report typical symptoms of CTS (according to the BCTQ), and the other 19 patients predominantly complained about mild symptoms. In contrast, 49 patients showed typical clinical signs of diabetic polyneuropathy (due to the NSS and NDS).

Electrodiagnostic testing is the technical gold standard to evaluate CTS [7]. It has been shown that approximately one quarter of diabetic patients had an electrophysiological, but clinically asymptomatic CTS while only 7.7% also had CTS symptoms [25]. A more recent study [14] found about 6.8% of persons with diabetes showing typical electrophysiological signs of CTS being clinically asymptomatic. Thus, it was suggested that asymptomatic CTS constellation in nerve conduction studies in diabetic patients are related to increased vulnerability of peripheral nerves at entrapment sites [14].

In our study, half of the patients showed a pathological increase in DML according to the cut-off values in our lab. Referring to the Bland classification [23] of electrophysiological severity of CTS, 37 patients met the diagnosis criteria for CTS and six patients were classified as severe or extremely severe. Thus, many more patients met the electrophysiological criteria for CTS diagnosis, while considerably fewer patients reported typical symptoms. The major hallmark of our study was that nerve conduction study was not able to differentiate between diabetic patients with CTS symptoms from diabetic patients without.

However, we did not use additional nerve conduction studies to increase sensitivity such as comparison studies of sensory-latency difference between the 2nd and 5th digit, between the median and ulnar part of the 4th digit, or between the median and radial thumb [26], which may be of additional value in diabetic patients.

Considering the results of peripheral nerve ultrasound in our study, the median nerve CSA at the wrist was larger than 12 mm^2 in 45 patients, and the wrist-to-forearm-ratio was larger than 1.4 in 61 patients.

It has been suggested before that sonographic assessment for the diagnosis of CTS requires a different cut-off value for diabetic patients [27]. A cut-off value for CSA of the median nerve at the wrist to diagnose coexisting CTS and diabetic polyneuropathy of 11.6 mm^2 was suggested (in contrast to the cut-off used for the diagnosis of CTS in nondiabetic patients of 9.2 mm^2) [28]. Others suggested a cut-off value of CSA at the wrist for CTS confirmation of more than 13 mm^2 in both diabetic and nondiabetic patients [29]. Overall, the cut-off values for CSA abnormality in CTS vary considerably in different studies and no consensus exists on a specific optimum cut-off value [9].

Nevertheless, ultrasound measurements in our study were not able to differentiate between patients with CTS symptoms and patients without, and even not between patients with polyneuropathy and those without.

A recent meta-analysis [15] of CSAs of the median nerve at the wrist level described larger CSA measurements in patient groups with both CTS and diabetes than in patients with CTS only and patients with diabetes only, and the smallest CSAs in normal controls. The wrist-to-forearm-ratio in CTS patients with diabetes was significantly lower than in nondiabetic patients, and no difference between the wrist-to-forearm-ratio could be demonstrated between diabetics with and without CTS [30]. It was suggested that an increase in median nerve CSA without change in the wrist-to-forearm-ratio might be an indicator of diabetic polyneuropathy [31]. However, this assumption could not be verified in our study.

In a study of patients with typical clinical symptoms of CTS, patients with diabetes tended to have a longer latency, smaller amplitude, and lower conduction velocity in nerve conduction studies compared to patients without diabetes mellitus, but the ultrasound CSA values did not differ significantly [32]. In contrast, it was found in a comparison between diabetic patients with symptomatic and asymptomatic CTS that the symptoms of CTS in patients with diabetes are related to CSA of the median nerve [33].

In a small percentage of patients with median nerve entrapment at the carpal tunnel, the CSA is abnormal at the outlet rather than the inlet of the carpal tunnel. However, we measured the CSA at the inlet only. CSA measurements at the outlet had possibly shown other results. In addition, other promising ultrasound techniques were not used in this study—particularly, the evaluation of echogenicity, the intraneural blood flow using Doppler ultrasound [9], or ultrasound elastography—to assess changes in stiffness of the nerve [34,35]. These techniques may provide additional information for CTS diagnosis but need more clinical evaluation.

Polyneuropathy is a common complication in diabetes mellitus [20]. In our study population, 49 (out of 69) patients had polyneuropathic symptoms. However, diabetic polyneuropathy causes alterations in nerve conduction studies [36,37] and in peripheral nerve ultrasound as well [27,38,39]. Generally, diabetic polyneuropathy leads to an enlargement of peripheral nerve CSAs with particular nerve enlargement at entrapment sites [27,40]. These sonographic alterations are explicitly less pronounced than those found in demyelinating polyneuropathies [41,42].

The presence of diabetic polyneuropathy has been shown to be associated with an increase in CSA of the median nerve at the carpal tunnel [16,31]. In contrast, others found median nerve CSA at the wrist significantly smaller in patients with CTS and diabetic polyneuropathy compared with diabetic patients with CTS only [15,43].

We found a correlation between distal motor latency and median nerve CSA at the wrist and also between distal motor latency and wrist-to-forearm-ratio, which shows that sonographically enlarged nerves also have slower conduction velocities. This was already shown generally in polyneuropathy [42,44] but also in CTS measurements in patients with diabetic neuropathy [45]. Moreover, it demonstrates that the measurements in our study show the same physiological relationship as those found in other studies and, therefore, seem conclusive. Nevertheless, NCS is generally seen to be superior to ultrasound for the identification of superimposed CTS in diabetic polyneuropathy [45,46].

Besides the existence of polyneuropathy, there may be additional factors able to influence carpal tunnel measurements. In our cohort, we found a small but significant influence of body mass index on median nerve CSA and HbA_{1c} on wrist-to-forearm-ratio. It has been shown that CTS was significantly associated with high body mass index in diabetic patients [47] and generally in the normal population also [48,49]. In addition, higher levels of HbA_{1c} and plasma glucose levels were shown to be associated with an increased risk for CTS in diabetic patients [50]. This shows that the quality of long-term blood glucose control (measured by HbA_{1c}) has an impact on CTS ultrasound measurements and, therefore, should be taken into account. It has to be noted that body mass index and HbA_{1c} also have a strong correlation to each other [51,52].

Limitations of the study are the relatively small sample size and the single-center character of the study. All patients were cared for in a tertiary care outpatient clinic for diabetology, which may introduce some selection bias towards patients with potentially more complicated diabetes mellitus. In addition, the study was not primarily designed to study CTS in diabetes. If electrodiagnostic testing and ultrasound had been conducted on the most symptomatic wrist, the results would possibly have been different. However, BCTQ scores were not strikingly different between the left and right hand. Nevertheless, strengths of the study are the use of standardized scores for CTS and diabetic neuropathy in addition to standardized electrophysiological and ultrasound measurements.

5. Conclusions

In conclusion, the major finding of our study was that neither the distal motor latency of the median nerve, the cross-sectional area of the median nerve at the wrist, nor the wrist-to-forearm-ratio were able to distinguish between diabetic patients with and without CTS symptoms. This may especially be caused as electrodiagnostic testing and peripheral nerve ultrasound of the carpal tunnel in diabetic patients may significantly be altered due to the existence of additional factors such as diabetic neuropathy, but also body mass index, hyperglycemia, and others. Therefore, it is advisable to primarily rely upon typical symptoms and clinical signs of CTS in diabetic patients. Results of electrodiagnostic testing and peripheral nerve ultrasound have to be interpreted with caution and additional factors have to be considered, especially the existence of diabetic polyneuropathy.

Author Contributions: Conceptualization, B.H., N.M., C.K. and H.A.; methodology, B.H. and H.A.; validation, H.A. and A.G.; formal analysis, H.A. and B.H.; investigation, B.H., L.I.E.E.W. and N.J.K.; resources, B.H.; data curation, B.H.; writing—original draft preparation, H.A. and B.H.; writing—review and editing, A.G., N.M., C.K., L.I.E.E.W. and N.J.K.; visualization, H.A.; project administration, B.H. and H.A. All authors have read and agreed to the published version of the manuscript.

Funding: This work was funded by the Deutsche Forschungsgemeinschaft (DFG, German Research Foundation) Clinician Scientist Program OrganAge funding number 413668513 and by the Interdisciplinary Center of Clinical Research of the Medical Faculty Jena.

Institutional Review Board Statement: This study was carried out in accordance with the Declaration of Helsinki. The study was approved by the local ethics committee (ethics committee of the Friedrich-Schiller-University Jena, number 2019-1416-BO).

Informed Consent Statement: All participants gave written informed consent.

Data Availability Statement: The data used to support the findings of this study are available from the corresponding author upon request.

Conflicts of Interest: The authors declare no conflict of interest. The funders had no role in the design of the study; in the collection, analyses, or interpretation of data; in the writing of the manuscript, or in the decision to publish the results.

References

1. Zimmerman, M.; Gottsäter, A.; Dahlin, L.B. Carpal Tunnel Syndrome and Diabetes—A Comprehensive Review. *J. Clin. Med.* **2022**, *11*, 1674. [CrossRef] [PubMed]
2. De Krom, M.C.; Kester, A.D.; Knipschild, P.G.; Spaans, F. Risk Factors for Carpal Tunnel Syndrome. *Am. J. Epidemiol.* **1990**, *132*, 1102–1110. [CrossRef] [PubMed]
3. Gül Yurdakul, F.; Bodur, H.; Öztop Çakmak, Ö.; Ateş, C.; Sivas, F.; Eser, F.; Yılmaz Taşdelen, Ö. On the Severity of Carpal Tunnel Syndrome: Diabetes or Metabolic Syndrome. *J. Clin. Neurol.* **2015**, *11*, 234–240. [CrossRef] [PubMed]
4. Chen, L.-H.; Li, C.-Y.; Kuo, L.-C.; Wang, L.-Y.; Kuo, K.N.; Jou, I.-M.; Hou, W.-H. Risk of Hand Syndromes in Patients with Diabetes Mellitus: A Population-Based Cohort Study in Taiwan. *Medicine* **2015**, *94*, e1575. [CrossRef] [PubMed]
5. Doughty, C.T.; Bowley, M.P. Entrapment Neuropathies of the Upper Extremity. *Med. Clin. N. Am.* **2019**, *103*, 357–370. [CrossRef]
6. Padua, L.; Coraci, D.; Erra, C.; Pazzaglia, C.; Paolasso, I.; Loreti, C.; Caliandro, P.; Hobson-Webb, L.D. Carpal Tunnel Syndrome: Clinical Features, Diagnosis, and Management. *Lancet Neurol.* **2016**, *15*, 1273–1284. [CrossRef]
7. Sasaki, T.; Koyama, T.; Kuroiwa, T.; Nimura, A.; Okawa, A.; Wakabayashi, Y.; Fujita, K. Evaluation of the Existing Electrophysiological Severity Classifications in Carpal Tunnel Syndrome. *J. Clin. Med.* **2022**, *11*, 1685. [CrossRef]
8. Pugdahl, K.; Tankisi, H.; Fuglsang-Frederiksen, A. Electrodiagnostic Testing of Entrapment Neuropathies: A Review of Existing Guidelines. *J. Clin. Neurophysiol.* **2020**, *37*, 299–305. [CrossRef]
9. Pelosi, L.; Arányi, Z.; Beekman, R.; Bland, J.; Coraci, D.; Hobson-Webb, L.D.; Padua, L.; Podnar, S.; Simon, N.; van Alfen, N.; et al. Expert Consensus on the Combined Investigation of Carpal Tunnel Syndrome with Electrodiagnostic Tests and Neuromuscular Ultrasound. *Clin. Neurophysiol.* **2022**, *135*, 107–116. [CrossRef]
10. Cartwright, M.S.; Hobson-Webb, L.D.; Boon, A.J.; Alter, K.E.; Hunt, C.H.; Flores, V.H.; Werner, R.A.; Shook, S.J.; Thomas, T.D.; Primack, S.J.; et al. Evidence-Based Guideline: Neuromuscular Ultrasound for the Diagnosis of Carpal Tunnel Syndrome. *Muscle Nerve* **2012**, *46*, 287–293. [CrossRef]
11. Walker, F.O.; Cartwright, M.S.; Alter, K.E.; Visser, L.H.; Hobson-Webb, L.D.; Padua, L.; Strakowski, J.A.; Preston, D.C.; Boon, A.J.; Axer, H.; et al. Indications for Neuromuscular Ultrasound: Expert Opinion and Review of the Literature. *Clin. Neurophysiol.* **2018**, *129*, 2658–2679. [CrossRef] [PubMed]
12. Hobson-Webb, L.D.; Massey, J.M.; Juel, V.C.; Sanders, D.B. The Ultrasonographic Wrist-to-Forearm Median Nerve Area Ratio in Carpal Tunnel Syndrome. *Clin. Neurophysiol.* **2008**, *119*, 1353–1357. [CrossRef] [PubMed]
13. Perkins, B.A.; Olaleye, D.; Bril, V. Carpal Tunnel Syndrome in Patients with Diabetic Polyneuropathy. *Diabetes Care* **2002**, *25*, 565–569. [CrossRef] [PubMed]
14. Kim, W.K.; Kwon, S.H.; Lee, S.H.; Sunwoo, I.N. Asymptomatic Electrophysiologic Carpal Tunnel Syndrome in Diabetics: Entrapment or Polyneuropathy. *Yonsei Med. J.* **2000**, *41*, 123–127. [CrossRef]
15. Chen, I.-J.; Chang, K.-V.; Lou, Y.-M.; Wu, W.-T.; Özçakar, L. Can Ultrasound Imaging Be Used for the Diagnosis of Carpal Tunnel Syndrome in Diabetic Patients? A Systemic Review and Network Meta-Analysis. *J. Neurol.* **2020**, *267*, 1887–1895. [CrossRef]
16. Attah, F.A.; Asaleye, C.M.; Omisore, A.D.; Kolawole, B.A.; Aderibigbe, A.S.; Alo, M. Relationship between Sonographically Measured Median Nerve Cross-Sectional Area and Presence of Peripheral Neuropathy in Diabetic Subjects. *World J. Diabetes* **2019**, *10*, 47–56. [CrossRef]
17. Levine, D.W.; Simmons, B.P.; Koris, M.J.; Daltroy, L.H.; Hohl, G.G.; Fossel, A.H.; Katz, J.N. A Self-Administered Questionnaire for the Assessment of Severity of Symptoms and Functional Status in Carpal Tunnel Syndrome. *J. Bone Joint Surg. Am.* **1993**, *75*, 1585–1592. [CrossRef]
18. Keilani, M.Y.; Pernicka, E.; Paternostro-Sluga, T.; Sycha, T.; Schett, G.; Pieber, K.; Fialka-Moser, V.; Crevenna, R. Übersetzung und Validierung des "Boston Carpal Tunnel Syndrome Questionnaire" zum Einsatz bei deutschsprachigen Patienten. *Phys. Med. Rehab. Kurortmed.* **2008**, *18*, 136–144. [CrossRef]
19. Young, M.J.; Boulton, A.J.; MacLeod, A.F.; Williams, D.R.; Sonksen, P.H. A Multicentre Study of the Prevalence of Diabetic Peripheral Neuropathy in the United Kingdom Hospital Clinic Population. *Diabetologia* **1993**, *36*, 150–154. [CrossRef]
20. Ziegler, D.; Keller, J.; Maier, C.; Pannek, J. Diabetic Neuropathy. *Exp. Clin. Endocrinol. Diabetes* **2021**, *129*, S70–S81. [CrossRef]
21. Stöhr, M.; Pfister, R. *Klinische Elektromyographie und Neurographie—Lehrbuch und Atlas*, 6th ed.; Kohlhammer: Stuttgart, Germany, 2014; pp. 397–399.

22. Linehan, C.; Childs, J.; Quinton, A.E.; Aziz, A. Ultrasound Parameters to Identify and Diagnose Carpal Tunnel Syndrome. A Review of the Literature. *Australas. J. Ultrasound Med.* **2020**, *23*, 194–206. [CrossRef] [PubMed]
23. Bland, J.D. A Neurophysiological Grading Scale for Carpal Tunnel Syndrome. *Muscle Nerve* **2000**, *23*, 1280–1283. [CrossRef]
24. Atroshi, I.; Gummesson, C.; Johnsson, R.; Ornstein, E.; Ranstam, J.; Rosén, I. Prevalence of Carpal Tunnel Syndrome in a General Population. *JAMA* **1999**, *282*, 153–158. [CrossRef]
25. Dyck, P.J.; Kratz, K.M.; Karnes, J.L.; Litchy, W.J.; Klein, R.; Pach, J.M.; Wilson, D.M.; O'Brien, P.C.; Melton, L.J.; Service, F.J. The Prevalence by Staged Severity of Various Types of Diabetic Neuropathy, Retinopathy, and Nephropathy in a Population-Based Cohort: The Rochester Diabetic Neuropathy Study. *Neurology* **1993**, *43*, 817–824. [CrossRef]
26. Alanazy, M.H. Clinical and Electrophysiological Evaluation of Carpal Tunnel Syndrome: Approach and Pitfalls. *Neurosciences* **2017**, *22*, 169–180. [CrossRef]
27. Kang, S.; Kim, S.H.; Yang, S.N.; Yoon, J.S. Sonographic Features of Peripheral Nerves at Multiple Sites in Patients with Diabetic Polyneuropathy. *J. Diabetes Complic.* **2016**, *30*, 518–523. [CrossRef] [PubMed]
28. Kim, L.-N.; Kwon, H.-K.; Moon, H.-I.; Pyun, S.-B.; Lee, H.-J. Sonography of the Median Nerve in Carpal Tunnel Syndrome with Diabetic Neuropathy. *Am. J. Phys. Med. Rehabil.* **2014**, *93*, 897–907. [CrossRef] [PubMed]
29. Tsai, N.-W.; Lee, L.-H.; Huang, C.-R.; Chang, W.-N.; Wang, H.-C.; Lin, Y.-J.; Lin, W.-C.; Lin, T.-K.; Cheng, B.-C.; Su, Y.-J.; et al. The Diagnostic Value of Ultrasonography in Carpal Tunnel Syndrome: A Comparison between Diabetic and Non-Diabetic Patients. *BMC Neurol.* **2013**, *13*, 65. [CrossRef]
30. Steinkohl, F.; Loizides, A.; Gruber, L.; Karpf, M.; Mörsdorf, G.; Gruber, I.; Glodny, B.; Löscher, W.; Gruber, H. Ultrasonography for the Diagnosis of Carpal Tunnel Syndrome in Diabetic Patients: Missing the Mark? *Rofo* **2019**, *191*, 117–121. [CrossRef]
31. Moon, H.I.; Kwon, H.K.; Kim, L.; Lee, H.J.; Lee, H.J. Ultrasonography of Palm to Elbow Segment of Median Nerve in Different Degrees of Diabetic Polyneuropathy. *Clin. Neurophysiol.* **2014**, *125*, 844–848. [CrossRef]
32. Kim, Y.H.; Yang, K.S.; Kim, H.; Seok, H.Y.; Lee, J.H.; Son, M.H.; Kim, B.J. Does Diabetes Mellitus Influence Carpal Tunnel Syndrome? *J. Clin. Neurol.* **2017**, *13*, 243–249. [CrossRef] [PubMed]
33. Han, H.Y.; Kim, H.M.; Park, S.Y.; Kim, M.-W.; Kim, J.M.; Jang, D.-H. Clinical Findings of Asymptomatic Carpal Tunnel Syndrome in Patients with Diabetes Mellitus. *Ann. Rehabil. Med.* **2016**, *40*, 489–495. [CrossRef] [PubMed]
34. Sung, J.H.; Kwon, Y.J.; Baek, S.-H.; Son, M.H.; Lee, J.H.; Kim, B.-J. Utility of Shear Wave Elastography and High-Definition Color for Diagnosing Carpal Tunnel Syndrome. *Clin. Neurophysiol.* **2022**, *135*, 179–187. [CrossRef]
35. Liu, F.; Li, D.; Xin, Y.; Liu, F.; Li, W.; Zhu, J. Quantification of Nerve Viscosity Using Shear Wave Dispersion Imaging in Diabetic Rats: A Novel Technique for Evaluating Diabetic Neuropathy. *Korean J. Radiol.* **2022**, *23*, 237–245. [CrossRef] [PubMed]
36. Padua, L.; Saponara, C.; Ghirlanda, G.; Padua, R.; Aprile, I.; Caliandro, P.; Tonali, P. Lower Limb Nerve Impairment in Diabetic Patients: Multiperspective Assessment. *Eur. J. Neurol.* **2002**, *9*, 69–73. [CrossRef]
37. Dunnigan, S.K.; Ebadi, H.; Breiner, A.; Katzberg, H.D.; Lovblom, L.E.; Perkins, B.A.; Bril, V. Conduction Slowing in Diabetic Sensorimotor Polyneuropathy. *Diabetes Care* **2013**, *36*, 3684–3690. [CrossRef]
38. Agirman, M.; Yagci, I.; Leblebicier, M.A.; Ozturk, D.; Akyuz, G.D. Is Ultrasonography Useful in the Diagnosis of the Polyneuropathy in Diabetic Patients? *J. Phys. Ther. Sci.* **2016**, *28*, 2620–2624. [CrossRef]
39. Watanabe, T.; Ito, H.; Sekine, A.; Katano, Y.; Nishimura, T.; Kato, Y.; Takeda, J.; Seishima, M.; Matsuoka, T. Sonographic Evaluation of the Peripheral Nerve in Diabetic Patients: The Relationship between Nerve Conduction Studies, Echo Intensity, and Cross-Sectional Area. *J. Ultrasound Med.* **2010**, *29*, 697–708. [CrossRef]
40. Ma, X.; Li, T.; Du, L.; Liu, G.; Sun, T.; Han, T. Applicability of High-Frequency Ultrasound to the Early Diagnosis of Diabetic Peripheral Neuropathy. *Biomed Res. Int.* **2021**, *2021*, 5529063. [CrossRef]
41. Grimm, A.; Vittore, D.; Schubert, V.; Rasenack, M.; Décard, B.F.; Heiling, B.; Hammer, N.; Axer, H. Ultrasound Aspects in Therapy-Naive CIDP Compared to Long-Term Treated CIDP. *J. Neurol.* **2016**, *263*, 1074–1082. [CrossRef]
42. Grimm, A.; Heiling, B.; Schumacher, U.; Witte, O.W.; Axer, H. Ultrasound Differentiation of Axonal and Demyelinating Neuropathies. *Muscle Nerve* **2014**, *50*, 976–983. [CrossRef] [PubMed]
43. Kotb, M.A.; Bedewi, M.A.; Aldossary, N.M.; Mahmoud, G.; Naguib, M.F. Sonographic Assessment of Carpal Tunnel Syndrome in Diabetic Patients with and without Polyneuropathy. *Medicine* **2018**, *97*, e11104. [CrossRef] [PubMed]
44. Di Pasquale, A.; Morino, S.; Loreti, S.; Bucci, E.; Vanacore, N.; Antonini, G. Peripheral Nerve Ultrasound Changes in CIDP and Correlations with Nerve Conduction Velocity. *Neurology* **2015**, *84*, 803–809. [CrossRef]
45. Drăghici, N.C.; Tămaș, M.M.; Leucuța, D.C.; Lupescu, T.D.; Strilciuc, Ș.; Rednic, S.; Mureșanu, D.F. Diagnosis Accuracy of Carpal Tunnel Syndrome in Diabetic Neuropathy. *Medicina* **2020**, *56*, 279. [CrossRef]
46. Hassan, A.; Leep Hunderfund, A.N.; Watson, J.; Boon, A.J.; Sorenson, E.J. Median Nerve Ultrasound in Diabetic Peripheral Neuropathy with and without Carpal Tunnel Syndrome. *Muscle Nerve* **2013**, *47*, 437–439. [CrossRef]
47. Bekele, A.; Abebe, G.; Hailu, T.; Fekadu, T.; Gebremickael, A.; Getachew, T.; Churko, C.; Alelign, D.; Wassihun, B.; Teshome, D.; et al. Prevalence and Associated Factors of Carpal Tunnel Syndrome Among Diabetic Patients in Arba Minch General Hospital, South West Ethiopia, 2021. *Diabetes Metab. Syndr. Obes.* **2022**, *15*, 983–993. [CrossRef] [PubMed]
48. Lampainen, K.; Shiri, R.; Auvinen, J.; Karppinen, J.; Ryhänen, J.; Hulkkonen, S. Weight-Related and Personal Risk Factors of Carpal Tunnel Syndrome in the Northern Finland Birth Cohort 1966. *J. Clin. Med.* **2022**, *11*, 1510. [CrossRef]

49. Wiberg, A.; Smillie, R.W.; Dupré, S.; Schmid, A.B.; Bennett, D.L.; Furniss, D. Replication of Epidemiological Associations of Carpal Tunnel Syndrome in a UK Population-Based Cohort of over 400,000 People. *J. Plast. Reconstr. Aesthet. Surg.* **2022**, *75*, 1034–1040. [CrossRef] [PubMed]
50. Rydberg, M.; Zimmerman, M.; Gottsäter, A.; Nilsson, P.M.; Melander, O.; Dahlin, L.B. Diabetes Mellitus as a Risk Factor for Compression Neuropathy: A Longitudinal Cohort Study from Southern Sweden. *BMJ Open Diabetes Res. Care* **2020**, *8*, e001298. [CrossRef]
51. Boye, K.S.; Lage, M.J.; Thieu, V.; Shinde, S.; Dhamija, S.; Bae, J.P. Obesity and Glycemic Control among People with Type 2 Diabetes in the United States: A Retrospective Cohort Study Using Insurance Claims Data. *J. Diabetes Complic.* **2021**, *35*, 107975. [CrossRef]
52. Ngiam, K.Y.; Lee, W.-J.; Lee, Y.-C.; Cheng, A. Efficacy of Metabolic Surgery on HbA1c Decrease in Type 2 Diabetes Mellitus Patients with BMI < 35 kg/m^2—A Review. *Obes. Surg.* **2014**, *24*, 148–158. [CrossRef] [PubMed]

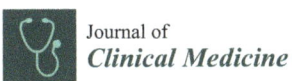

Article

Correlation between Electrodiagnostic Study and Imaging Features in Patients with Suspected Carpal Tunnel Syndrome

Jae Min Song [1], Jungyun Kim [1], Dong-Jin Chae [1], Jong Bum Park [1], Yung Jin Lee [1], Cheol Mog Hwang [2], Jieun Shin [3] and Mi Jin Hong [1,*]

1. Department of Rehabilitation Medicine, Konyang University College of Medicine, Daejeon 35365, Korea; green4leaf@naver.com (J.M.S.); kirshna0615@hanmail.net (J.K.); coehdwls@hanmail.net (D.-J.C.); jbocean@hanmail.net (J.B.P.); eutravel@kyuh.ac.kr (Y.J.L.)
2. Department of Radiology, Konyang University College of Medicine, Daejeon 35365, Korea; rad@kyuh.ac.kr
3. Department of Biomedical Informatics, Konyang University College of Medicine, Daejeon 35365, Korea; jeshin@konyang.ac.kr
* Correspondence: yvvvyvvvy@gmail.com; Tel.: +82-42-612-2187

Abstract: Electrodiagnostic studies (EDXs) are the confirmative diagnostic tool for carpal tunnel syndrome (CTS). Previous studies have evaluated the relationship between EDXs and ultrasonography (US) but not with X-rays. Recently, many studies on the diagnostic value of X-rays in various diseases have been reported, but data on CTS are lacking. We evaluated the relationship between electrodiagnostic parameters and roentgenographic and ultrasonographic features in CTS and investigated the usefulness of X-rays and US for CTS. This retrospective study included 97 wrists of 62 patients. All patients with suspected CTS underwent EDXs, wrist US, and wrist X-rays. The CTS patients were classified into mild, moderate, and severe groups. The roentgenographic features included the ulnar variance (UV) and the anteroposterior diameter of the wrist (APDW), and the ultrasonographic features included the flattening ratio (FR) and the thickest anteroposterior diameter of the median nerve (TAPDM). Most EDX parameters showed significant correlations with roentgenographic and US features. The electrodiagnostic severity was also correlated with all imaging features. Therefore, both wrist X-rays and wrist US can be useful for the diagnosis of CTS as supplements to EDXs.

Keywords: carpal tunnel syndrome; electrodiagnosis; X-rays; ultrasonography; median nerve

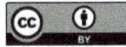

1. Introduction

Carpal tunnel syndrome (CTS), or entrapment neuropathy of the median nerve at the wrist, is a common condition associated with numbness, tingling, pain that frequently worsens at night, and atrophy in the thenar region as the typical symptoms [1]. Thus, a patient with these symptoms is considered to have CTS, and women are much more apt to have this condition than men [2].

Electrodiagnostic studies (EDXs) are the confirmative diagnostic tool and are also used for severity grading, but they do not provide anatomic information at the wrist. Therefore, ultrasonography (US) has been used to visualize the median nerve and its surrounding anatomic structures [3,4]. Several studies have been conducted on various US features useful for the diagnosis of CTS, including the cross-sectional area (CSA), flattening ratio (FR), palmar bowing, thickest anteroposterior diameter of the median nerve (TAPDM), and the wrist-to-forearm ratio [4–10]. However, it is still unknown which one is the most indicative of CTS. Buchberger et al. [6] first reported that compared to normal wrists, the median nerves of CTS patients were significantly flattened. Duncan et al. [7] revealed significant differences in the FR of the median nerve and the TAPDM between CTS patients and controls.

There have been insufficient studies showing that simple X-rays have a diagnostic value for CTS, but they have the advantage of providing morphological images easily and inexpensively. Considerable progress in the development of radiology technology has been made, and studies on the diagnostic value of X-rays have recently been reported [11]. Among five roentgenographic features, Ikeda et al. [12] reported that there was a statistically significant difference in ulnar variance (UV) between CTS patients and controls. Therefore, additional research on the usefulness of plain radiography for the diagnosis of CTS is required.

A few other studies have evaluated the relationship between EDXs and US features. However, to our knowledge, no study has evaluated the relationship between EDXs and roentgenographic features. Therefore, we were interested in (1) examining the relationship between EDX parameters and roentgenographic and US features in patients with suspected CTS and (2) confirming the usefulness of roentgenographic and US features as a tool for diagnosing CTS.

2. Materials and Methods

2.1. Subjects

This study was designed as a retrospective chart review. We collected the data of 68 patients between January 2019 and May 2021. The patients who visited the outpatient department of rehabilitation medicine in a single center with some or all symptoms of CTS and underwent EDXs, wrist US, and wrist simple X-rays were selected for the study. The symptoms were sensory abnormalities in median nerve distribution, nocturnal pain, atrophy in the thenar region, and several positive provocative tests (Tinel sign, Phalen's maneuver, and reverse Phalen's maneuver) [13–15]. The exclusion criteria were as follows: (1) Patients with a history of wrist surgery or injections and any upper extremity trauma; (2) patients with neurologic diseases, such as diabetic polyneuropathy, brachial plexopathy, ulnar neuropathy, proximal median neuropathy (entrapment of the ligament of Struthers, pronator syndrome, anterior interosseous nerve syndrome), cervical radiculopathy, and rheumatic diseases; and (3) patients with hereditary or metabolic diseases that can cause peripheral neuropathy. Six patients were excluded due to insufficient wrist images. Finally, 97 wrists of 62 patients were enrolled in this study (Figure 1). The study was approved by the Institutional Review Board of Konyang University College of Medicine (IRB no. 2021-06-010).

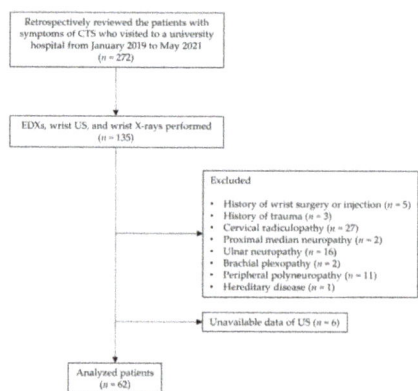

Figure 1. Study flow chart. Abbreviations: CTS, carpal tunnel syndrome; EDXs, electrodiagnostic studies; US, ultrasonography.

2.2. Electrodiagnostic Studies

EDXs were conducted using Natus Synergy on a Nicolet EDX machine. All patients underwent needle electromyography and routine nerve conduction studies (NCSs) with an antidromic technique, including median and ulnar NCSs [16]. The temperature of both hands was measured and maintained between 32 °C to 34 °C. For the sensory NCS of the median nerve, a surface ground electrode was placed over the dorsum of the hand. A pair of surface recording electrodes were placed in line over the index finger at an inter-electrode distance of 4 cm. Standard stimulation was conducted at two sites that were 14 cm proximal to the active electrode (wrist) and 7 cm proximal to the active electrode (palm). For the motor NCS of the median nerve, the belly-tendon method was used for recording. A surface ground electrode was placed over the same site as that used in the sensory NCS. A surface active electrode was placed over the center of the belly of the abductor pollicis brevis (APB) muscle, and a surface reference electrode was placed distally over the tendon of the APB muscle. Standard supramaximal stimulation was conducted at the wrist. The sensory NCS parameters collected were the onset latency, peak latency, baseline-to-peak amplitude, and conduction velocity. The motor NCS parameter collected was the distal motor latency.

When the routine NCS results were normal, we performed three additional Preston's median-versus-ulnar comparison studies [17]. In the palmar mixed comparison study, the median mixed nerve latency across the palm was compared to the adjacent ulnar mixed nerve latency using identical distances between the stimulation and recording sites. In the digit 4 comparison study, the median sensory latency recording of digit 4 was compared to the ulnar sensory latency recording of digit 4, using identical distances between the stimulation and recording sites. In the lumbrical-interossei comparison study, the median motor latency recording of the second lumbrical was compared to the ulnar motor latency recording of the interossei using identical distances between the stimulation and recording sites. A very mild CTS score (grade 1 on the Bland scale) was assigned when two or more of these three sensitive studies were positive.

The severity of the patients was classified according to the Bland scale using the EDX results [18]. Grade 0 (normal) indicated no neurophysiological abnormality in the sensory and motor conduction studies. Grade 1 (very mild CTS) indicated that abnormalities were detected in two or more sensitive tests. Grade 2 (mild CTS) indicated slowing sensory nerve conduction velocity and normal distal motor latency (<4.5 ms from the wrist to the APB muscle). Grade 3 (moderately severe CTS) indicated preserved sensory potential and slowing distal motor latency (>4.5 ms and <6.5 ms). Grade 4 (severe CTS) indicated absent sensory potential and slowing distal motor latency (>4.5 ms and <6.5 ms). Grade 5 (very severe CTS) indicated absent sensory potential and slowing distal motor latency (>6.5 ms), and grade 6 (extremely severe CTS) indicated decreased surface motor potential from the APB (<0.2 mV).

The above severity grades were also reclassified into four severity groups [19]. A severity grade of 0 was the control group, severity grades 1 and 2 were classified as the mild group; a severity grade of 3 was assigned to the moderate group; and severity grades of 4, 5, and 6 were classified as the severe group (Table 1).

Table 1. Reclassification of severity grade by electrodiagnostic study.

Severity Grade *	Severity Group
0	Control
1	Mild
2	
3	Moderate
4	Severe
5	
6	

* Severity grades of 0–6 according to the Bland scale.

2.3. Wrist X-rays

All patients underwent simple X-rays of the posteroanterior and lateral view of the wrist. To obtain the posteroanterior view, the elbow was flexed 90°, the forearm was pronated, and the wrist was in a neutral position. The UV was defined as the distance between horizontal lines (that were perpendicular to the long axis of the radius/ulna) drawn from the distal ulnar and radial articular surfaces (at the level of the distal radioulnar joint) on a posteroanterior view (Figure 2A) [12,20]. To obtain the lateral view, the elbow was flexed 90° and adducted against the trunk, and the wrist was in a neutral position. The anteroposterior diameter of the wrist (APDW) was defined as the distance between the volar and dorsal edge of the distal radius on a lateral view (Figure 2B) [12]. Two raters performed the measurements without other information on the patients, and the mean of the measurements was used in the analyses.

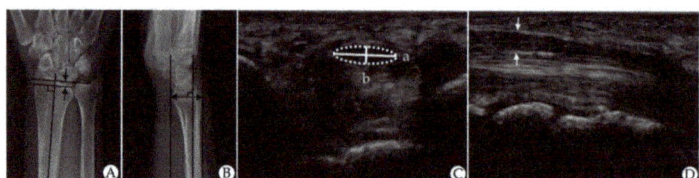

Figure 2. Measurements of ultrasonographic and roentgenographic features. (**A**) Ulnar variance on X-rays (the distance between the two arrows). (**B**) AP diameter of the wrist on X-rays (the distance of the arrow). (**C**) Flattening ratio on US (a (width)/b (height)). (**D**) Thickest AP diameter of the median nerve on US (the distance between the two arrows). Abbreviations: AP, anteroposterior; US, ultrasonography.

2.4. Ultrasonography

An experienced radiologist who was blinded to all of the patient's results conducted the US evaluations using an ultrasound system with a 5–15 MHz linear transducer (GE LOGIQ E9; General Electrical Healthcare, China). No additional force was applied other than the weight of the probe. The FR of the median nerve was calculated as the ratio of the nerve's major axis to its minor axis at the pisiform bone level on the transverse view (a/b) (Figure 2C) [7]. The TAPDM, including the hypoechogenic median nerve and hyperechogenic nerve sheath, was measured between the carpal tunnel inlet and outlet on the longitudinal view (Figure 2D) [9]. Two raters performed the measurements without other information on the patients, and the mean of the measurements was used in the analyses.

2.5. Statistical Analyses

Statistical analyses were performed using SPSS statistical software version 28.0 for Windows (IBM, Armonk, NY, USA). First, to examine differences in the distribution of demographic characteristics, we used the chi-square test for categorical variables and the analysis of variance (ANOVA) for continuous variables. Second, Pearson's correlation coefficient was used to assess the relationship between EDXs and roentgenographic features, EDXs and US features, and roentgenographic and US features. Because sensory potentials were absent in the severe group and could not be quantified, the correlation analysis could not include the severe group, so the analysis included all except the severe group. Third, to examine differences in roentgenographic and ultrasonographic features in CTS patients and controls, we used *t*-test. Furthermore, to examine differences in roentgenographic and ultrasonographic features between the four severity groups, we used one-way ANOVA. If the result of ANOVA was statistically significant, Scheffe's method was additionally used for multiple comparisons in post hoc analysis. Lastly, logistic regression analysis was conducted to evaluate the independent, related variables of CTS in the four imaging features and to determine the odds ratio (OR) and corresponding 95% confidence intervals (95% CI). Stepwise backward elimination was used to identify the most significant predictor of CTS. The diagnostic value of the imaging features was evaluated by the area under the receiver operator characteristics (ROC) curve. All analyses were tested at the significance level of 0.05.

3. Results

3.1. Demographic Characteristics

The demographic characteristics of the subjects are shown in Table 2. The subjects were 17 males and 45 females. The mean ages of the participants in the four groups were 41.13 ± 14.46, 53.50 ± 9.05, 59.80 ± 8.43, and 62.89 ± 8.43 years, respectively. Age and sex were significantly different between the four groups, and the ratio of left hands to right hands was not significantly different.

Table 2. Demographic characteristics of the subjects.

		Control	Mild CTS	Moderate CTS	Severe CTS	p-Value
Number of Hands		30	34	15	18	
Age (years)		41.13 ± 14.46	53.50 ± 9.05	59.80 ± 8.43	62.89 ± 8.43	<0.001
Sex	Male	11	2	4	6	0.021
	Female	19	32	11	12	
Side	Right	14	20	8	10	0.806
	Left	16	14	7	8	

Values are presented as the mean ± standard deviation. Abbreviation: CTS, carpal tunnel syndrome.

3.2. Relationship between Electrodiagnostic Parameters and Roentgenographic and Ultrasonographic Features

Pearson's correlation coefficient is shown in Tables 3 and 4. First, both the UV and APDW, which were roentgenographic features, showed statistically significant correlations with all EDX parameters, except for between UV and distal motor latency. Second, the FR and TAPDM showed statistically significant correlations with all EDX parameters. Especially, the correlation coefficients between sensory onset latency and the FR ($r = 0.772$), sensory peak latency and the FR ($r = 0.772$), sensory conduction velocity and the FR ($r = -0.725$), and distal motor latency and the FR ($r = 0.703$) were relatively high. Third, there were significant relationships between all roentgenographic features and all US features.

Table 3. Pearson's correlation coefficients between electrodiagnostic parameters and imaging features.

EDXs	X-ray		Ultrasonography	
	UV	APDW	FR	TAPDM
Sensory onset latency	0.358 **	0.333 **	0.772 ***	0.458 ***
Sensory peak latency	0.334 **	0.332 **	0.772 ***	0.438 ***
Sensory amplitude	−0.443 ***	−0.428 ***	−0.652 ***	−0.370 **
Sensory conduction velocity	−0.361 **	−0.357 **	−0.725 ***	−0.488 ***
Distal motor latency	0.139	0.306 **	0.703 ***	0.434 ***

** $p < 0.01$, *** $p < 0.001$. Abbreviations: EDXs, electrodiagnostic studies; UV, ulnar variance; APDW, AP diameter of the wrist; FR, flattening ratio; TAPDM, thickest AP diameter of the median nerve.

Table 4. Pearson's correlation coefficient between ultrasonographic and roentgenographic features.

		X-ray		Ultrasonography	
		UV	APDW	FR	TAPDM
X-ray	UV	1			
	APDW	0.310 **	1		
Ultrasonography	FR	0.320 **	0.467 ***	1	
	TAPDM	0.283 *	0.391 ***	0.320 **	1

* $p < 0.05$, ** $p < 0.01$, *** $p < 0.001$. Abbreviations: UV, ulnar variance; APDW, AP diameter of the wrist; FR, flattening ratio; TAPDM, thickest AP diameter of the median nerve.

3.3. Differences in Roentgenographic and Ultrasonographic Features between CTS Patients and Controls

The imaging features in the CTS patients and controls are summarized in Table 5. There were significant differences in all four imaging features between the two groups. The mean UV was 1.45 ± 1.89 in the CTS patients and -0.01 ± 1.55 in the controls. The mean APDW was 23.81 ± 2.34 mm in the CTS patients and 22.14 ± 2.07 mm in the controls. The mean FR was 3.53 ± 0.52 in the CTS patients and 2.81 ± 0.28 in the controls. The mean TAPDM was 2.44 ± 0.46 mm in the CTS patients and 1.97 ± 0.35 mm in the controls.

Table 5. Roentgenographic and ultrasonographic features in CTS patient and control groups.

	Control Group	CTS Patient Group	*p*-Value
UV	-0.01 ± 1.55	1.45 ± 1.89	<0.001
APDW (mm)	22.14 ± 2.07	23.81 ± 2.34	0.001
FR	2.81 ± 0.28	3.53 ± 0.52	<0.001
TAPDM (mm)	1.97 ± 0.35	2.44 ± 0.46	<0.001

Values are presented as the mean ± standard deviation. Abbreviations: UV, ulnar variance; APDW, AP diameter of the wrist; FR, flattening ratio; TAPDM, thickest AP diameter of the median nerve.

3.4. Differences in Roentgenographic and Ultrasonographic Features between the Four Severity Groups

The roentgenographic and the US features in the four severity groups are shown in Table 6. The mean UV and standard deviation were -0.01 ± 1.55, 1.69 ± 2.18, 0.96 ± 1.61, and 1.41 ± 1.61 in the control, mild, moderate, and severe groups, respectively. The APDW was 22.14 ± 2.07 mm, 23.11 ± 2.29 mm, 23.85 ± 1.93 mm, and 25.09 ± 1.93 mm, respectively. The FR was 2.81 ± 0.28, 3.24 ± 0.41, 3.80 ± 0.48, and 3.87 ± 0.48, respectively. The TAPDM was 1.97 ± 0.35 mm, 2.34 ± 0.39 mm, 2.49 ± 0.52 mm, and 2.58 ± 0.52 mm, respectively. All imaging features showed statistically significant differences.

Table 6. Roentgenographic and ultrasonographic features in four severity groups.

	Control Group	Mild Group	Moderate Group	Severe Group	*p*-Value
UV	-0.01 ± 1.55 [c]	1.69 ± 2.18	0.96 ± 1.61	1.41 ± 1.61 [c]	0.003
APDW (mm)	22.14 ± 2.07 [b]	23.11 ± 2.29	23.85 ± 1.93 [b]	25.09 ± 1.93	<0.001
FR	2.81 ± 0.28 [a, b, c]	3.24 ± 0.41 [a, d, e]	3.80 ± 0.48 [b, d]	3.87 ± 0.48 [c, e]	<0.001
TAPDM (mm)	1.97 ± 0.35 [a, b, c]	2.34 ± 0.39 [a]	2.49 ± 0.52 [b]	2.58 ± 0.52 [c]	<0.001

Values are presented as the mean ± standard deviation. In post-hoc analysis, [a] $p < 0.05$ in control group vs. mild group, [b] $p < 0.05$ in control group vs. moderate group, [c] $p < 0.05$ in control group vs. severe group, [d] $p < 0.05$ in mild group vs. moderate group, and [e] $p < 0.05$ in mild group vs. severe group. Abbreviations: UV, ulnar variance; APDW, AP diameter of the wrist; FR, flattening ratio; TAPDM, thickest AP diameter of the median nerve.

Scheffe's multiple comparison test was conducted for post hoc analysis. There was a significant difference in UV between the control and severe groups. There was a significant difference in APDW between the control and moderate groups. In the FR, there were significant differences between all subgroups except for the moderate and severe groups. There were significant differences in the TAPDM between the control and all CTS groups.

3.5. Factors Related to Carpal Tunnel Syndrome

The OR and 95% CI in univariate logistic regression of the four imaging features adjusted for baseline age values are presented in Table 7. Neither UV ($p = 0.05$, OR 1.43, 95% CI 1.00–2.04) nor APDW ($p = 0.237$, OR 1.16, 95% CI 0.91–1.48) were significantly related to CTS. However, the FR ($p < 0.001$, OR 86.52, 95% CI 9.26–808.83) and the TAPDM ($p < 0.002$, OR 15.33, 95% CI 2.78–84.62) were significantly associated with CTS. The ROC curves are shown in Figure 3. The area under the curve (AUC) of the UV and the APDW was 0.832 ($p < 0.001$) and 0.805 ($p < 0.001$), respectively. The AUC of the FR and the TAPDM was 0.927 ($p < 0.001$) and 0.889 ($p < 0.001$), respectively. Table 7 also shows the multiple logistic regression analysis results using backward elimination. The FR ($p = 0.001$, OR 52.52, 95% CI 5.50–501.73) and the TAPDM ($p = 0.032$, OR 8.91, 95% CI 1.20–65.97) were significant variables, so they remained in the model.

Table 7. Univariate logistic regression analysis and multiple logistic regression analysis using stepwise backward elimination.

	Univariate Logistic Regression				Multiple Logistic Regression			
	Odds Ratio	95% Confidence Interval		p-Value	Odds Ratio	95% Confidence Interval		p-Value
		Lower	Upper			Lower	Upper	
UV	1.43	1	2.04	0.05				
APDW	1.16	0.91	1.48	0.237				
FR	86.52	9.26	808.83	<0.001	52.52	5.5	501.73	0.001
TAPDM	15.33	2.78	84.62	0.002	8.91	1.2	65.97	0.032

Abbreviations: UV, ulnar variance; APDW, AP diameter of the wrist; FR, flattening ratio; TAPDM, thickest AP diameter of the median nerve.

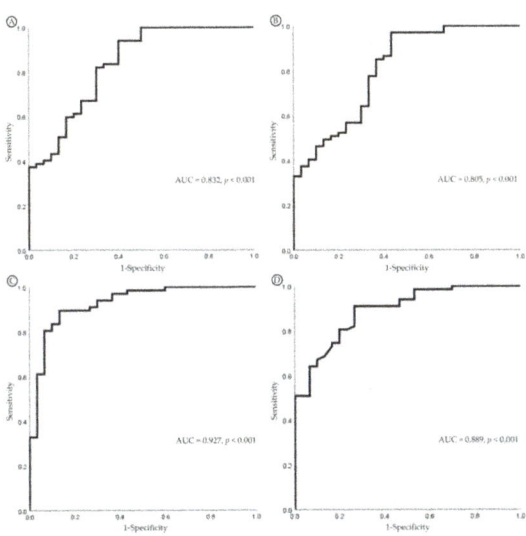

Figure 3. Receiver operating characteristic (ROC) curves for the diagnosis of CTS. (**A**) UV. (**B**) APDW. (**C**) FR. (**D**) TAPDM. Abbreviations: CTS, carpal tunnel syndrome; UV, ulnar variance; APDW, AP diameter of the wrist; FR, flattening ratio; TAPDM, thickest AP diameter of the median nerve; AUC, area under the curve.

4. Discussion

EDXs have been widely used as the standard test for diagnosing CTS. Routine NCS or various comparison studies [21] can confirm electrophysiologic abnormalities of the median nerve within the carpal tunnel and the location of the lesion can be confirmed using the inching technique [22]. However, due to the disadvantage of not being able to obtain information on the anatomic structure of the wrist along with pain experienced during the examination, several imaging tests, including magnetic resonance imaging (MRI), computed tomography (CT), US, and X-rays, have been used together. Among them, both the US and X-rays have the common advantages of being easy, fast, non-invasive, and painless for the patient during the examination. Buchberger et al. [5,6] first reported the usefulness of US features such as the CSA, FR, and palmar bowing for CTS based on wrist MRIs, and Ikeda et al. [12] revealed the usefulness of roentgenographic features for CTS. However, they did not investigate the relationship between imaging features and various EDX parameters, which is the difference and uniqueness between this study and other previous studies. Our study demonstrated that all EDX parameters were correlated with all roentgenographic and US features, with just one exception between distal motor latency and the UV. In the post hoc analysis (Table 6), there was a significant difference in UV only between the control group and the severe group. Therefore, excluding the severe group from the correlation analysis could have caused this result. The sensory onset latency and sensory peak latency showed positive correlations with all imaging features, and the sensory amplitude and sensory conduction velocity showed negative correlations with all imaging features.

The UV represents the relative length of the ulna compared to the radius [23]. Cha et al. [24] reported a significant relationship between a decreased CSA around the distal radioulnar joint and a positive UV in CTS patients, supporting the importance of a positive UV in the development of CTS. Our UV findings were consistent with those of Ikeda et al. [12]. CTS patients showed a significantly high UV value compared to the controls. This finding suggests that although UV refers to the state of the extra space in the carpal tunnel and does not directly impact the median nerve, an imbalance in the distal radioulnar joint may be involved in the development of CTS [12,24].

The APDW is a popular and simple measurement of wrist size, estimating the carpal tunnel size. Carpal tunnel size has been a controversial risk factor for CTS. Bleecker et al. [25] and Dekel et al. [26] found that the carpal tunnel was smaller in CTS patients than in controls. Conversely, Winn et al. [27] reported that CTS patients had a larger carpal tunnel area than matched controls. Uchiyama et al. [28] showed that the proximal and distal carpal tunnel areas were significantly larger in mild-to-moderate and severe CTS patient groups than in the control group except for the extreme CTS group. The results of our study were similar. The APDW was larger in CTS patients than in the controls. Considering both the above findings, we suggest that there are other anthropometric risk factors or work-related factors, and further studies are needed.

Various studies have confirmed localized swelling and flattening of the median nerve in CTS patients by US or MRI [5,6,29,30]. Duncan et al. [7] reported an FR of 3.2 in CTS patients and 2.7 in controls by US at the level of the pisiform bone, which is usually the level of the maximum swelling of the median nerve. Additionally, they reported a TAPDM of 2.2 mm in CTS patients and 1.8 mm in controls by US. Uchiyama et al. [28] showed that the FR was significantly larger at the pisiform bone level in the mild-to-moderate, severe, and extreme CTS groups than in the control group based on MRI. Kim et al. [9] revealed that there were statistical differences in the TAPDM between CTS patients and controls. Likewise, we revealed that the FR and TAPDM values in CTS patients were larger than in the controls. Therefore, we also confirmed the swelling and flattening of the median nerve in CTS patients.

Identifying the factors related to CTS can be helpful in diagnosing CTS more precisely. The logistic regression analysis results showed that two US features were significantly related to CTS, and a higher FR was the most predictive factor for CTS. We speculate that this was due to the advantage of US, which can directly show the swelling and flattening of the median nerve. As reported in other studies, we also found that the US features could be useful for diagnosing CTS. Notably, the results of our study confirmed that the roentgenographic features were correlated with the EDXs and US features, and there was a significant difference between the CTS patient group and the control group. X-rays have limitations in that they mainly show bony structures and cannot show vascularity and tendons. However, they also have several advantages. They are relatively inexpensive compared to other imaging studies, and if they are conducted according to an accurate position and protocol, X-rays can be a more objective test than US, which can be relatively subjective depending upon the examiner.

This study had some limitations that should be considered. First, the retrospective nature was a major limitation. Due to the lack of data, we could not include information on CTS risk factors, such as the body mass index, wrist circumference, and participant occupation. This may have limited the generalizability of the results. Second, there were relatively fewer subjects, a higher percentage of female patients, and this was a single-center study. Particularly, the sample size of the control patients was small, and they were relatively young. Thus, these factors may have affected the logistic regression analysis, yielding a relatively high OR and wide 95% CI range. However, the fact that CTS occurs more frequently in women and between the ages of 50 and 60 should be taken into account. Third, although it is known that age affects nerve conduction velocity and waveform morphology, there were significant differences in age between the four groups. To compensate for this, we adjusted for baseline age values in the logistic regression analysis. Finally, no inter-rater reliability test was performed. However, two raters performed the measurements, and the average of the measured values was used. Despite these limitations, to our knowledge, this was the first study to report associations between EDXs and roentgenographic features. Further studies with a larger number of subjects are necessary to confirm and generalize our findings.

5. Conclusions

This study showed that most EDX parameters were correlated with roentgenographic and ultrasonographic features, and the electrodiagnostic severity was correlated with all wrist imaging features. Although the US features showed statistically better results than the roentgenographic features, depending upon the situation, X-rays can also be useful for diagnosing CTS. Therefore, we recommend considering both wrist X-rays and wrist US for patients with CTS symptoms to supplement EDXs. This will make the diagnosis of CTS more accurate. Furthermore, a larger follow-up study is necessary to reinforce the clinical effectiveness of wrist X-rays in CTS.

Author Contributions: Conceptualization, M.J.H., J.B.P. and Y.J.L.; investigation, J.M.S. and M.J.H.; resources, J.M.S., J.K., D.-J.C. and C.M.H.; data curation, J.S.; writing—original draft preparation, J.M.S.; writing—review and editing, M.J.H. All authors have read and agreed to the published version of the manuscript.

Funding: This research received no external funding.

Institutional Review Board Statement: This study was approved by the Institutional Review Board of Konyang University College of Medicine (IRB no. 2021-06-010).

Informed Consent Statement: Patient consent was waived because of the study's retrospective design.

Data Availability Statement: The datasets used and/or analyzed in this study are available from the corresponding author upon reasonable request.

Conflicts of Interest: The authors declare no conflict of interest.

References

1. Dawson, D.M. Entrapment neuropathies of the upper extremities. *N. Engl. J. Med.* **1993**, *329*, 2013–2018. [CrossRef] [PubMed]
2. Phalen, G.S. The carpal-tunnel syndrome. Clinical evaluation of 598 hands. *Clin. Orthop. Relat. Res.* **1972**, *83*, 29–40. [CrossRef] [PubMed]
3. Jablecki, C.K.; Andary, M.T.; So, Y.T.; Wilkins, D.E.; Williams, F.H. Literature review of the usefulness of nerve conduction studies and electromyography for the evaluation of patients with carpal tunnel syndrome. AAEM Quality Assurance Committee. *Muscle Nerve* **1993**, *16*, 1392–1414. [PubMed]
4. Wong, S.M.; Griffith, J.F.; Hui, A.C.; Lo, S.K.; Fu, M.; Wong, K.S. Carpal tunnel syndrome: Diagnostic usefulness of sonography. *Radiology* **2004**, *232*, 93–99. [CrossRef]
5. Buchberger, W.; Schön, G.; Strasser, K.; Jungwirth, W. High-resolution ultrasonography of the carpal tunnel. *J. Ultrasound Med.* **1991**, *10*, 531–537. [CrossRef]
6. Buchberger, W.; Judmaier, W.; Birbamer, G.; Lener, M.; Schmidauer, C. Carpal tunnel syndrome: Diagnosis with high-resolution sonography. *AJR Am. J. Roentgenol.* **1992**, *159*, 793–798. [CrossRef]
7. Duncan, I.; Sullivan, P.; Lomas, F. Sonography in the diagnosis of carpal tunnel syndrome. *AJR Am. J. Roentgenol.* **1999**, *173*, 681–684. [CrossRef]
8. Ferrari, F.S.; Della Sala, L.; Cozza, S.; Guazzi, G.; Belcapo, L.; Mariottini, A.; Bolognini, A.; Stefani, P. High-resolution ultrasonography in the study of carpal tunnel syndrome. *Radiol. Med.* **1997**, *93*, 336–341.
9. Kim, H.J.; Lee, B.N. Correlation of Ultrasonography with the Nerve Conduction Study in Carpal Tunnel Syndrome of Koreans. *J. Korean Assoc. EMG Electrodiagn. Med.* **2006**, *8*, 21–25.
10. Hobson-Webb, L.D.; Massey, J.M.; Juel, V.C.; Sanders, D.B. The ultrasonographic wrist-to-forearm median nerve area ratio in carpal tunnel syndrome. *Clin. Neurophysiol.* **2008**, *119*, 1353–1357. [CrossRef]
11. Adams, S.J.; Henderson, R.D.E.; Yi, X.; Babyn, P. Artificial Intelligence Solutions for Analysis of X-ray Images. *Can. Assoc. Radiol. J.* **2021**, *72*, 60–72. [CrossRef] [PubMed]
12. Ikeda, K.; Yoshii, Y.; Ogawa, T.; Ishii, T. Radiographic characteristics of wrists in idiopathic carpal tunnel syndrome patients. *BMC Musculoskelet. Disord.* **2020**, *21*, 1–8. [CrossRef] [PubMed]
13. Stewart, J.; Eisen, A. Tinel's sign and the carpal tunnel syndrome. *Br. Med. J.* **1978**, *2*, 1125. [CrossRef] [PubMed]
14. Kuschner, S.H.; Ebramzadeh, E.; Johnson, D.; Brien, W.W.; Sherman, R. Tinel's sign and Phalen's test in carpal tunnel syndrome. *Orthopedics* **1992**, *15*, 1297–1302. [CrossRef]
15. Werner, R.A.; Bir, C.; Armstrong, T.J. Reverse Phalen's maneuver as an aid in diagnosing carpal tunnel syndrome. *Arch. Phys. Med. Rehabil.* **1994**, *75*, 783–786. [CrossRef]
16. Preston, D.C.; Shapiro, B.E. Routine upper extremity, facial, and phrenic nerve conduction techniques. In *Electromyography and Neuromuscular Disorders E-Book: Clinical-Electrophysiologic-Ultrasound Correlations*, 4th ed.; Elsevier Health Sciences: Amsterdam, The Netherlands, 2020; pp. 107–111.
17. Preston, D.C.; Shapiro, B.E. Median neuropathy at the wrist. In *Electromyography and Neuromuscular Disorders E-Book: Clinical-Electrophysiologic-Ultrasound Correlations*, 4th ed.; Elsevier Health Sciences: Amsterdam, The Netherlands, 2020; pp. 329–331.
18. Bland, J.D. A neurophysiological grading scale for carpal tunnel syndrome. *Muscle Nerve Off. J. Am. Assoc. Electrodiagn. Med.* **2000**, *23*, 1280–1283. [CrossRef]
19. Mohammadi, A.; Ghasemi-Rad, M.; Mladkova-Suchy, N.; Ansari, S. Correlation between the severity of carpal tunnel syndrome and color Doppler sonography findings. *Am. J. Roentgenol.* **2012**, *198*, W181–W184. [CrossRef]
20. Lalone, E.A.; Grewal, R.; King, G.J.; MacDermid, J.C. A structured review addressing the use of radiographic measures of alignment and the definition of acceptability in patients with distal radius fractures. *Hand* **2015**, *10*, 621–638. [CrossRef]
21. Werner, R.A.; Andary, M. Electrodiagnostic evaluation of carpal tunnel syndrome. *Muscle Nerve* **2011**, *44*, 597–607. [CrossRef]
22. Kang, Y.K.; Kim, D.H.; Lee, S.H.; Hwang, M.; Han, M.S. Tenelectrodes: A new stimulator for inching technique in the diagnosis of carpal tunnel syndrome. *Yonsei Med. J.* **2003**, *44*, 479–484. [CrossRef]
23. De Smet, L. Ulnar variance: Facts and fiction review article. *Acta Orthop. Belg.* **1994**, *60*, 1–9. [PubMed]
24. Cha, S.M.; Shin, H.D.; Song, S.H. Cross-sectional Area Just Proximal to the Carpal Tunnel According to the Ulnar Variances: Positive Ulnar Variance and Carpal Tunnel Syndrome. *Ann. Plast. Surg.* **2019**, *82*, 76–81. [CrossRef] [PubMed]
25. Bleecker, M.L.; Bohlman, M.; Moreland, R.; Tipton, A. Carpal tunnel syndrome: Role of carpal canal size. *Neurology* **1985**, *35*, 1599. [CrossRef] [PubMed]
26. Dekel, S.; Papaioannou, T.; Rushworth, G.; Coates, R. Idiopathic carpal tunnel syndrome caused by carpal stenosis. *Br. Med. J.* **1980**, *280*, 1297–1299. [CrossRef] [PubMed]
27. Winn Jr, F.J.; Habes, D.J. Carpal tunnel area as a risk factor for carpal tunnel syndrome. *Muscle Nerve Off. J. Am. Assoc. Electrodiagn. Med.* **1990**, *13*, 254–258. [CrossRef]
28. Uchiyama, S.; Itsubo, T.; Yasutomi, T.; Nakagawa, H.; Kamimura, M.; Kato, H. Quantitative MRI of the wrist and nerve conduction studies in patients with idiopathic carpal tunnel syndrome. *J. Neurol. Neurosurg. Psychiatry* **2005**, *76*, 1103–1108. [CrossRef]
29. Mesgarzadeh, M.; Schneck, C.D.; Bonakdarpour, A.; Mitra, A.; Conaway, D. Carpal tunnel: MR imaging. Part II. Carpal tunnel syndrome. *Radiology* **1989**, *171*, 749–754. [CrossRef]

30. Middleton, W.; Kneeland, J.; Kellman, G.; Cates, J.; Sanger, J.; Jesmanowicz, A.; Froncisz, W.; Hyde, J. MR imaging of the carpal tunnel: Normal anatomy and preliminary findings in the carpal tunnel syndrome. *Am. J. Roentgenol.* **1987**, *148*, 307–316. [CrossRef]

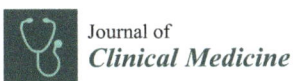

Article

Evaluation of the Existing Electrophysiological Severity Classifications in Carpal Tunnel Syndrome

Toru Sasaki [1,2], Takafumi Koyama [1], Tomoyuki Kuroiwa [1], Akimoto Nimura [3], Atsushi Okawa [1], Yoshiaki Wakabayashi [4] and Koji Fujita [3,*]

[1] Department of Orthopaedic and Spinal Surgery, Graduate School of Medical and Dental Sciences, Tokyo Medical and Dental University, 1-5-45, Yushima, Bunkyo-ku, Tokyo 113-8519, Japan; t-sasaki.orth@tmd.ac.jp (T.S.); koya.orth@tmd.ac.jp (T.K.); kurorth@gmail.com (T.K.); okawa.orth@tmd.ac.jp (A.O.)

[2] Department of Orthopaedic Surgery, Tsuchiura Kyodo General Hospital, 4-1-1, Tsuchiura 300-0028, Ibaraki, Japan

[3] Department of Functional Joint Anatomy, Graduate School of Medical and Dental Sciences, Tokyo Medical and Dental University, 1-5-45, Yushima, Bunkyo-ku, Tokyo 113-8519, Japan; nimura.orj@tmd.ac.jp

[4] Department of Orthopaedic Surgery, Yokohama City Minato Red Cross Hospital, 3-12-1, Shinyamashita, Naka-ku, Yokohama City 231-8582, Kanagawa, Japan; dr_waka@cl.cilas.net

* Correspondence: fujiorth@tmd.ac.jp; Tel.: +81-3-5803-5279

Abstract: Electrophysiological examination is important for the diagnosis and evaluation of nerve function in carpal tunnel syndrome (CTS). Electrophysiological severity classifications of CTS using a nerve conduction study (NCS) have been reported, and there are many reports on the relationship between severity classifications and clinical symptoms. The existing electrophysiological severity classifications have several problems, such as cases that do not fit into a classification and unclear reasons for the boundary value. The purpose of this study was to clarify the relationship between sensory nerve conduction velocity (SCV) and distal motor latency (DML) and to evaluate whether the existing severity classification method is appropriate. We created a scatter diagram between SCV and DML for our NCSs and found a negative correlation between SCV and DML (correlation coefficient, −0.786). When we applied our NCSs to the existing classifications (Padua and Bland classifications), there were many unclassifiable cases (15.2%; Padua classification), and the number of Grade 3 cases was significantly higher than that of Grade 2 or 4 cases (Bland classification). Our large dataset revealed a strong negative correlation between SCV and DML, indicating that the existing severity classifications do not always accurately reflect the severity of the disease.

Keywords: carpal tunnel syndrome; nerve conduction study; median nerve; electrophysiological severity classification

Citation: Sasaki, T.; Koyama, T.; Kuroiwa, T.; Nimura, A.; Okawa, A.; Wakabayashi, Y.; Fujita, K. Evaluation of the Existing Electrophysiological Severity Classifications in Carpal Tunnel Syndrome. *J. Clin. Med.* **2022**, *11*, 1685. https://doi.org/10.3390/jcm11061685

Academic Editors: Christian Carulli and Michael Sauerbier

Received: 1 February 2022
Accepted: 16 March 2022
Published: 18 March 2022

Publisher's Note: MDPI stays neutral with regard to jurisdictional claims in published maps and institutional affiliations.

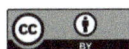

Copyright: © 2022 by the authors. Licensee MDPI, Basel, Switzerland. This article is an open access article distributed under the terms and conditions of the Creative Commons Attribution (CC BY) license (https://creativecommons.org/licenses/by/4.0/).

1. Introduction

Carpal tunnel syndrome (CTS) is identified by numbness, pain, and disordered thumb opposition associated with localized compression of the median nerve at the wrist and is the most common nerve entrapment syndrome [1–6]. Although CTS is diagnosed mainly based on clinical findings, an electrophysiological examination is important for diagnosis and determining the appropriate course of treatment [7–10]. Electrophysiological severity classification of CTS using a nerve conduction study (NCS) is a useful method that can easily display results of electrophysiological examination with several parameters on a single scale, and various classification methods have been reported [6,11–13]. In addition, there have been many reports on the assessment of clinical symptoms using electrophysiological severity classifications [14–17].

A previous study reported that because sensory fibers have a large proportion of large myelinated fibers, they are more susceptible to ischemic damage [6,18]. In clinical practice, numbness due to sensory disturbance is more likely to be recognized at an early stage than muscle atrophy due to motor disturbance [19,20]. Therefore, many existing severity classifications are based on the premise that CTS is a disorder of sensory fiber dominance [6,11–13]. However, motor nerve fiber damage appears long before the appearance of muscle atrophy, and sensory nerve damage does not necessarily occur first. The reasons for the boundary value that separates severities are not clear in the existing classifications, and we have had cases in which patient results do not fit the existing classifications. We thought it necessary to examine whether or not the existing severity classifications can accurately evaluate the degree of disability in CTS patients.

We hypothesized that the existing electrophysiological severity classifications have several problems such as the existence of cases that do not fit the classifications and unclear reasons for the boundary value. The purpose of this study was to determine the relationship between sensory nerve conduction velocity (SCV) and distal motor latency (DML) using data from NCSs on patients with CTS at our hospital and apply the NCS data to the existing severity classifications (Padua and Bland classifications) to evaluate whether the existing classifications are appropriate classification methods.

2. Materials and Methods

2.1. Participants

In this retrospective study, all clinical and NCS data were obtained from the 560 patients (1120 hands; median age, 69.5 years; 264 male hands, 856 female hands) treated at the department of orthopedic surgery at Tokyo Medical and Dental University (Table 1). We obtained written informed consent from all the participants. This retrospective analysis was approved by our institutional review board. This study included patients who were suspected of having CTS by hand surgeons and underwent NCSs between April 2007 and September 2019 at our hospital. The inclusion criteria for this study were as follows: clinical symptoms of CTS (numbness, tingling, and pain) and positive examination findings for CTS, including a positive Phalen test and Tinel's sign. In addition to the patients who underwent NCSs preoperatively, the patients who had CTS symptoms, underwent NCSs postoperatively, and had abnormal results were also included in this study. The patients whose symptoms disappeared after surgery and had normal SCV and DL were excluded. Since the purpose of the study was to electrophysiologically evaluate sensory and motor neuropathies at the carpal tunnel area, patients with peripheral polyneuropathy, cervical disease, de Quervain syndrome, or trigger finger and those with a history of a distal radial fracture were also included in this study. Although peripheral polyneuropathy and cervical disease may cause abnormal results in NCSs, we included them in our analysis. In addition, although patients with de Quervain syndrome or trigger finger and those with a history of a distal radial fracture may have wrist pain, numbness, and a positive Tinel's sign at the carpal tunnel, we included these patients. This is because the participants of this study were diagnosed by hand surgeons as having neuropathy in the carpal tunnel area, and the main neuropathy is considered to be entrapment of the median nerve in the carpal tunnel area even if there are other comorbidities. Patients were excluded from this study if they could not undergo NCSs due to pain caused by electrical stimulation.

Table 1. Characteristics of the participants.

	n = 1120 Hands
Age [1]	69.5 (60–77)
Sex Male Female	 132 patients, 264 hands 428 patients, 856 hands
Pre-operation	247 patients, 494 hands
Post-operation	313 patients, 626 hands
Measurable DML and measurable SCV	934 hands
Non-measurable DML and non-measurable SCV	62 hands

[1] Data are presented as the medians (interquartile range). Abbreviations: DML, distal motor latency; SCV, sensory nerve velocity.

2.2. Nerve Conduction Study

NCSs were performed on both hands of each patient by trained clinical technicians, with patients relaxed and in the supine position. A skin temperature of 32 °C was maintained on the dorsum of the hand. An NCS of both median nerves was performed using an evoked potential/electromyography system (MEB-2300; Nihon Kohden, Tokyo, Japan) with the bandpass filter set to 5–10 Hz for motor nerve recording and 2–20 Hz for sensory recording. The sensory nerve action potential of the median nerve was antidromically recorded with a pair of cup electrodes placed on the index finger. Square-pulse supramaximal electrical stimuli at 0.5 Hz with a duration of 0.3 ms were delivered to the palm, wrist, and elbow. We calculated the sensory nerve conduction velocity (SCV) from the latency of the waveform of the sensory nerve action potential and the distance between the stimulation point and the recording electrode. The compound muscle action potential was recorded with a pair of surface cup electrodes placed over the abductor pollicis brevis by using the belly–tendon method. Square-pulse supramaximal electrical stimuli at 0.5 Hz with a duration of 0.3 ms were delivered to the wrist and elbow. The wrist stimulation point was 7 cm proximal to the cathode electrode placed on the abductor pollicis brevis. Distal motor latency (DML) was determined from the waveform of the compound motor action potential. Each measurement was performed twice to confirm reproducibility. The neurologists and orthopedic surgeons calculated the SCV and DML values from the waveforms. Those with unclear latency and no reproducibility were considered non-measurable.

2.3. Analysis

First, we analyzed the relationship between SCV and DML from the 1120 right and left hands of 560 patients. The results of the NCSs on the healthy side were also included in the analysis. We created a scatter diagram to study the correlation between SCV and DML using data from 934 hands in which both SCV and DML were measurable. The correlation coefficient of this scatter diagram was calculated, and the relationship between SCV and DML was evaluated. Furthermore, only patients with diabetes were extracted, and a scatter diagram was created in the same way. We added an analysis that excluded patients with peripheral polyneuropathy or cervical disease and postoperative patients. We also created a scatter diagram for these patients.

The NCS results of 1120 hands were then applied to the existing severity classifications (Padua and Bland classifications). A six-level classification (Grades 1–6) was created in the Padua classification. The boundary values of SCV and DML were set to 44 m/s and 4.0 ms, respectively [12] (Figure 1a). In the Bland classification, a seven-level classification (Grades 0–6) was created. The boundary values of SCV and DML were set to 40 m/s and 4.5–6.5 ms, respectively [11] (Figure 1b). We counted the number of cases that could not fit these classifications and extracted the problems of these systems by applying the results of our NCSs to the two classifications.

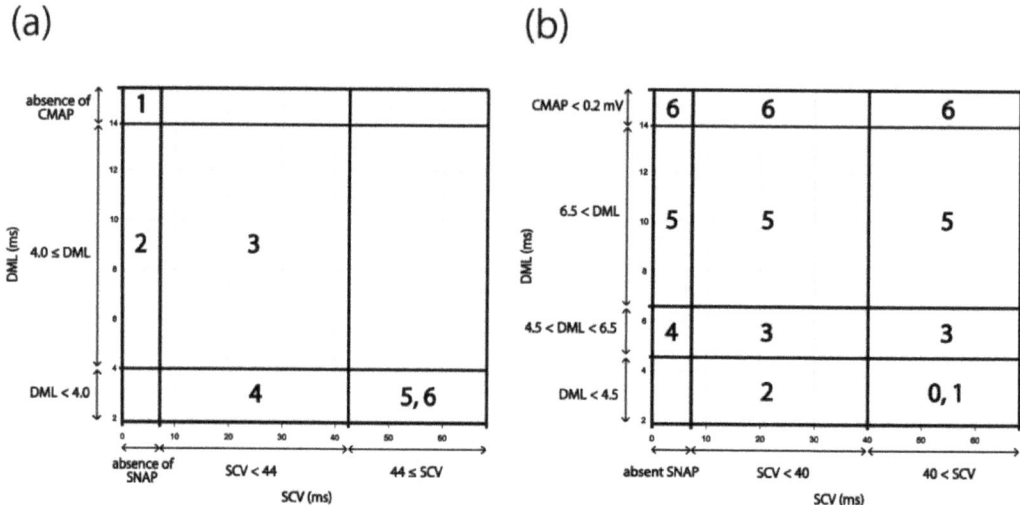

Figure 1. Electrophysiological severity classifications for CTS. (**a**) Padua classification. 1. Extreme CTS: absence of SNAP and CMAP. 2. Severe CTS: absence of SNAP and DML ≥ 4.0 ms. 3. Moderate CTS: SCV < 44 m/s and DML ≥ 4.0 ms. 4. Mild CTS: SCV < 44 m/s and DML < 4.0 ms. 5. Minimal CTS: "standard negative" hands with abnormal comparative or segmental tests. 6. Negative: normal findings on all tests. (**b**) Bland classification. Grade 0: no neurophysiological abnormalities. Grade 1: very mild CTS, detected only in two sensitivity tests (e.g., inching, palm/wrist median/ulnar comparison, ring finger "double peak"). Grade 2: mild CTS (SCV < 40 m/s and DML < 4.5 ms). Grade 3: moderately severe CTS (4.5 ms < DML < 6.5 ms and SCV < 40 m/s). Grade 4: severe CTS (4.5 ms < DML < 6.5 ms and absent SNAP). Grade 5: very severe CTS (6.5 ms < DML). Grade 6: extremely severe CTS (CMAP < 0.2 mV). Abbreviations: CMAP, compound muscle action potential; CTS, carpal tunnel syndrome; DML, distal motor latency; SCV, sensory nerve conduction velocity; SNAP, sensory nerve action potential.

3. Results

NCSs were performed on 1120 hands. The participants' demographic characteristics are presented in Table 1. There were 28 patients with diabetes (56 hands), 42 patients with cervical desease (84 hands), 60 patients with de Quervain syndrome or trigger finger (120 hands), and nine patients with a history of a distal radial fracture (18 hands). There were 247 preoperative patients (494 hands) and 313 postoperative patients (626 hands).

3.1. Relationship between SCV and DML

A scatter diagram was created using the results for 934 hands in which both SCV and DML were measurable. Both the SCV and DML values showed a strong negative correlation with a Spearman's rank correlation coefficient of −0.786 (Figure 2) [21,22]. The scatter diagram of diabetes patients also showed a strong negative correlation between SCV and DML (53 hands) (Spearman's rank correlation coefficient of −0.841) (Figure 3). The scatter diagram that excluded the patients with peripheral polyneuropathy or cervical disease and the postpoerative patients also showed a strong negative correlation between SCV and DML (320 hands) (Spearman's rank correlation coefficient of −0.779) (Figure 4).

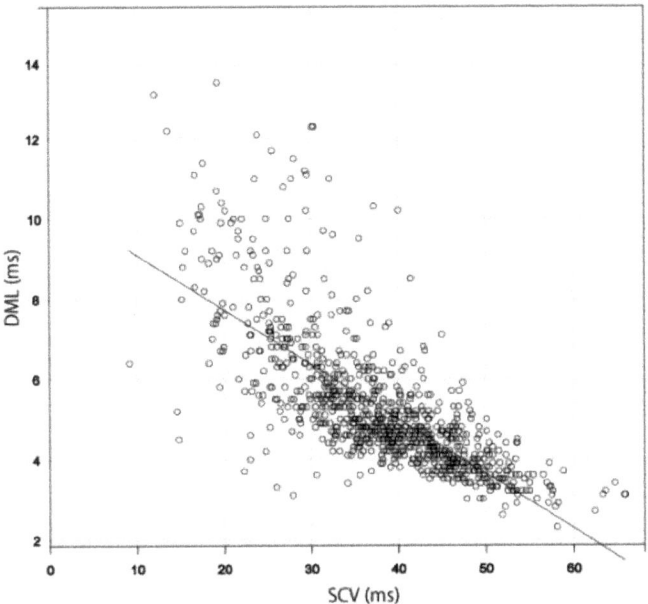

Figure 2. Scatter diagram between SCV and DML. The straight line shows the correlation between SCV and DML. Abbreviations: DML, distal motor latency; SCV, sensory nerve conduction velocity.

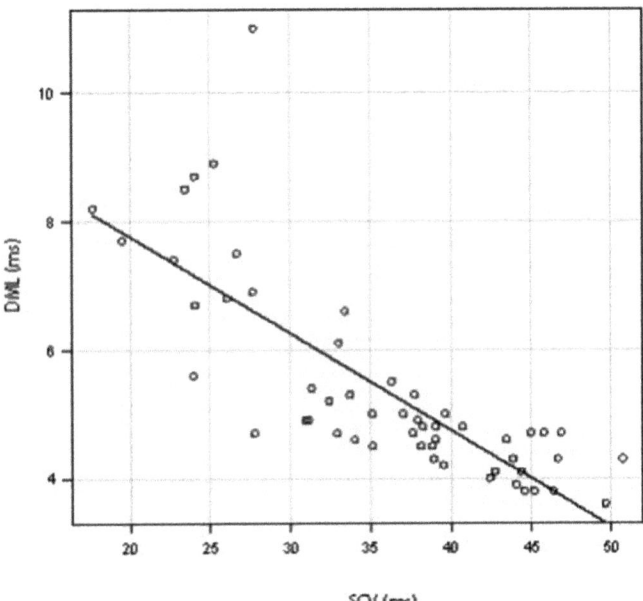

Figure 3. Scatter diagram between SCV and DML in the diabetes patients. The straight line shows the correlation between SCV and DML. Abbreviations: DML, distal motor latency; SCV, sensory nerve conduction velocity.

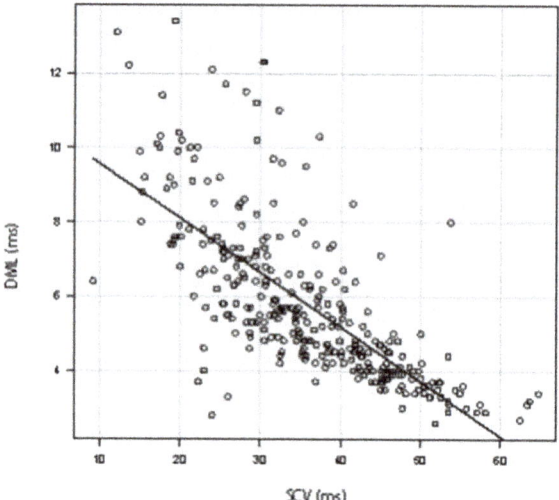

Figure 4. Scatter diagram between SCV and DML that excluded the patients with peripheral polyneuropathy or cervical disease and the postoperative patients. The straight line shows the correlation between SCV and DML. Abbreviations: DML, distal motor latency; SCV, sensory nerve conduction velocity.

3.2. Applying the Results to the Existing Severity Classifications

In the Padua classification, cases with normal SCV but abnormal DML and cases with measurable SCV but non-measurable DML were unclassifiable; thus, 170 of the 1120 cases (15.2%) could not be classified (Figure 5a). In the Bland classification, all the cases could be classified (Figure 5b), including 260 cases that were Grade 0 or 1, 59 cases that were Grade 2, 449 cases that were Grade 3, 10 cases that were Grade 4, 248 cases that were Grade 5, and 94 cases that were Grade 6. The number of Grade 3 cases was significantly higher than that of Grade 2 or 4 cases.

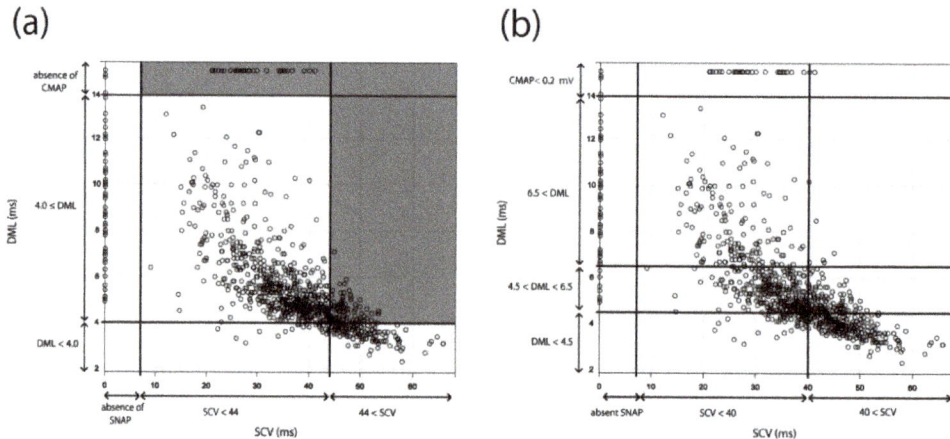

Figure 5. Results applied to the existing classifications. The NCS results of 1120 cases were applied to the existing severity classifications (Figure 1). (**a**) Padua classification: gray areas indicate cases that could not be classified. (**b**) Bland classification. Abbreviations: CMAP, compound muscle action potential; DML, distal motor latency; NCS, nerve conduction study; SCV, sensory nerve conduction velocity; SNAP, sensory nerve action potential.

4. Discussion

In this study, we showed that SCV and DML had a strong negative correlation using the NCS results of the CTS patients (all patients, diabetic patients, and patients who were excluded postoperatively) and those with peripheral polyneuropathy or cervical disease. We applied the results to the existing severity classification, and the following problems were identified: unclassifiable cases in the Padua classification and bias of the number in the Bland classification.

A previous study reported that because sensory fibers had a large proportion of large myelinated fibers, they were more susceptible to ischemic damage [6,18]; the Padua and Bland classifications were based on this premise [11,13]. However, our results show that SCV and DML have a strong negative correlation, indicating that we could not conclude whether the sensory fibers or motor fibers are damaged first. When our NCS results were applied to the existing severity classifications, 15.2% of cases could not be categorized using the Padua classification. Cases with normal SCV but abnormal DML and cases with measurable SCV but non-measurable DML were unclassifiable. The high number of unclassifiable cases was due to the fact that the Padua classification was based on sensory fiber dominance. Similarly, the Stevens and Werner classifications, which are cited in many papers, are based on the premise that sensory nerves are damaged first, and unclassifiable cases are also observed in these classifications [6,13]. According to previous reports, Martin–Gruber anastomosis (MGA) is present in 5–40% of patients, which may lead to prolonged DML and normal or higher SCV values [23]. Given the influence of MGA and our results suggesting that SCV and DML are strongly correlated, it may not be appropriate to use these classifications in clinical assessment.

Although all the results of NCSs were categorized in the Bland classification, as Bland himself states, a motor terminal latency measurement of 6.5 ms was arbitrary and the reasons for the boundary values (DML: 4.5, 6.5 ms, SCV: 4.0 m/s) were not clearly reported [11]. Furthermore, the Bland classification does not reflect the severity of disease in the order of classification. In the Bland classification, the cases in which sensory fibers were damaged first were classified as Grade 2 (area A of Figure 6), and those in which motor fibers were damaged first were classified as Grade 3 (area B of Figure 6). In other words, the cases in which motor fibers were damaged first were considered more severe in the Bland classification. However, motor and sensory fibers had a strong correlation in our results; thus, cases in area B were not necessarily more severe than those in area A (Figure 6). Furthermore, in Figure 6, the cases in areas B and C were classified as Grade 3 using the Bland classification. However, it is not necessarily correct to state that cases in areas B and C have the same severity because most cases in area C were more severe than those in area B when taking the correlation line into consideration. Because areas B and C were classified as having the same severity (Grade 3), the number of Grade 3 cases may have been notably higher than that of Grades 2 and 4 when using the Bland classification. Although Bland allows individual laboratories to define abnormal sensory and motor conduction values for Grades 2, 3, and 4, adjusting the definition for abnormal values will not solve this problem.

An electrophysiological study provides useful information for an objective and quantitative assessment of the neurophysiological severity of CTS [24–26]. Median nerve conduction studies in CTS cases evaluate both sensory and motor nerve fibers. Electrophysiological severity classification in CTS is a useful method to show these evaluation parameters on a single scale [11,12], and there are many reports on clinical evaluations using severity classifications [27–34]. However, as shown in this paper, the existing severity classifications do not always accurately reflect the severity of disease, and our results suggest the need to reevaluate previous studies that used these classifications.

There was a limitation in this study: we did not consider MGA in this study. As MGA can affect the results of NCS, patients with and without MGA should be analyzed separately for an accurate evaluation of the relationship between SCV and DML.

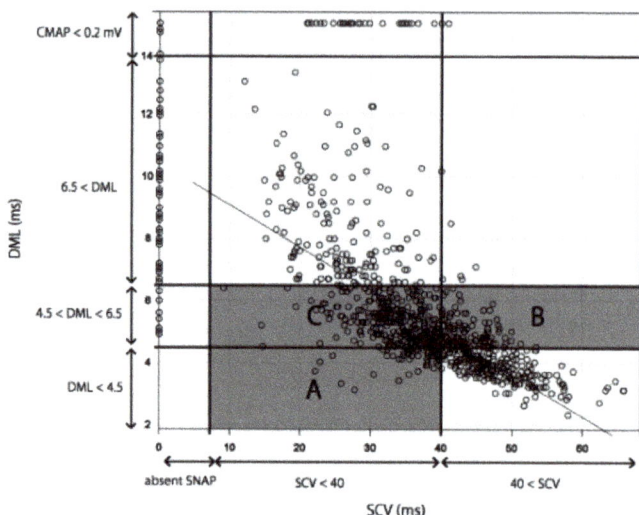

Figure 6. Analysis of the Bland classification. Area A: Grade 2 in Figure 1b. Area B: normal SCV in Grade 3 in Figure 1b. Area C: SCV < 40 m/s in Grade 3 in Figure 1b. The straight line shows the correlation between SCV and DML in Figure 2. Abbreviations: CMAP, compound muscle action potential; DML, distal motor latency; SCV, sensory nerve conduction velocity; SNAP, sensory nerve action potential.

In conclusion, our large dataset revealed a strong negative correlation between SCV and DML in our NCSs in patients with CTS. Problems with the existing severity classifications were higlighted, such as unclassifiable cases, unclear boundary values, different classifications for the same degree of severity, and the same classifications for different degrees of severity. In the future, it will be necessary to develop a comprehensive CTS severity classification that includes physical findings and subjective symptoms, while taking into account the correlation between sensory and motor fiber disorders.

Author Contributions: Conceptualization, T.S., K.F., A.O. and Y.W.; methodology, software, validation, formal analysis, visualization, supervision, T.S. and K.F.; investigation, resources, data curation, T.S., T.K. (Takafumi Koyama) and T.K. (Tomoyuki Kuroiwa); writing—original draft preparation, T.S. and K.F.; writing—review and editing, K.F. and A.N.; project administration, T.S. and K.F.; funding acquisition, K.F. All authors have read and agreed to the published version of the manuscript.

Funding: This work was funded by Japan Science and Technology Agency (JST) AIP-PRISM, grant No. JPMJCR18Y2.

Institutional Review Board Statement: The study was conducted in accordance with the Declaration of Helsinki and the protocol was approved in 2017 by the Institutional Review Board of Tokyo Medical and Dental University, approval No. M2017-108-01.

Informed Consent Statement: Informed consent was obtained from all the subjects involved in the study.

Data Availability Statement: The data generated in this study are available from the corresponding author on reasonable request.

Conflicts of Interest: The authors declare no conflict of interest. The funders had no role in the design of the study; in the collection, analyses, or interpretation of data; in the writing of the manuscript, or in the decision to publish the results.

References

1. Fujita, K.; Kimori, K.; Nimura, A.; Okawa, A.; Ikuta, Y. MRI analysis of carpal tunnel syndrome in hemodialysis patients versus non-hemodialysis patients: A multicenter case-control study. *J. Orthop. Surg. Res.* **2019**, *14*, 91. [CrossRef]
2. Jablecki, C.K.; Andary, M.T.; Floeter, M.K.; Miller, R.G.; Quartly, C.A.; Vennix, M.J.; Wilson, J.R. Practice parameter: Electrodiagnostic studies in carpal tunnel syndrome: Report of the American Association of Electrodiagnostic Medicine, American Academy of Neurology, and the American Academy of Physical Medicine and Rehabilitation. *Neurology* **2002**, *58*, 1589–1592. [CrossRef]
3. Kouyoumdjian, J.; Zanetta, D.M.; Morita, M.P. Evaluation of age, body mass index, and wrist index as risk factors for carpal tunnel syndrome severity. *Muscle Nerve* **2001**, *25*, 93–97. [CrossRef]
4. Kuroiwa, T.; Fujita, K.; Nimura, A.; Miyamoto, T.; Sasaki, T.; Okawa, A. A new method of measuring the thumb pronation and palmar abduction angles during opposition movement using a three-axis gyroscope. *J. Orthop. Surg. Res.* **2018**, *13*, 288. [CrossRef]
5. Kuroiwa, T.; Nimura, A.; Suzuki, S.; Sasaki, T.; Okawa, A.; Fujita, K. Measurement of thumb pronation and palmar abduction angles with a small motion sensor: A comparison with Kapandji scores. *J. Hand Surg.* **2019**, *44*, 728–733. [CrossRef]
6. Werner, R.A.; Andary, M. Electrodiagnostic evaluation of carpal tunnel syndrome. *Muscle Nerve* **2011**, *44*, 597–607. [CrossRef]
7. AAEM Quality Assurance Committee; Jablecki, C.K.; Andary, C.M.T.; So, Y.T.; Wilkins, D.E.; Williams, F.H. Literature review of the usefulness of nerve conduction studies and electromyography for the evaluation of patients with carpal tunnel syndrome. *Muscle Nerve* **1993**, *16*, 1392–1414. [CrossRef]
8. Nathan, P.A.; Keniston, R.C.; Meadows, K.D.; Lockwood, R.S. Predictive value of nerve conduction measurements at the carpal tunnel. *Muscle Nerve* **1993**, *16*, 1377–1382. [CrossRef]
9. Sonoo, M.; Menkes, D.L.; Bland, J.D.; Burke, D. Nerve conduction studies and EMG in carpal tunnel syndrome: Do they add value? *Clin. Neurophysiol. Pract.* **2018**, *3*, 78–88. [CrossRef]
10. You, H.C.; Simmons, Z.; Freivalds, A.; Kothari, M.J.; Naidu, S.H. Relationships Between Clinical Symptom Severity Scales and Nerve Conduction Measures in Carpal Tunnel Syndrome. *Muscle Nerve* **1999**, *22*, 497–501. [CrossRef]
11. Bland, J.D. A Neurophysiological Grading Scale for Carpal Tunnel Syndrome. *Muscle Nerve* **2000**, *23*, 1280–1283. [CrossRef]
12. Padua, L.; Lomonaco, M.; Gregori, B.; Valente, E.M.; Padua, R.; Tonali, P. Neurophysiological classification and sensitivity in 500 carpal tunnel syndrome hands. *Acta Neurol. Scand.* **2009**, *96*, 211–217. [CrossRef] [PubMed]
13. Stevens, J.C. AAEM Minimonograph #26: The Electrodiagnosis of Carpal Tunnel Syndrome. American Association of Electrodiagnostic Medicine. *Muscle Nerve* **1997**, *20*, 1477–1486. [CrossRef] [PubMed]
14. Aulisa, L.; Tamburrelli, F.; Padua, R.; Romanini, E.; Monaco, M.L.; Padua, L. Carpal tunnel syndrome: Indication for surgical treatment based on electrophysiologic study. *J. Hand Surg.* **1998**, *23*, 687–691. [CrossRef]
15. Bland, J.D. Do nerve conduction studies predict the outcome of carpal tunnel decompression? *Muscle Nerve* **2001**, *24*, 935–940. [CrossRef]
16. Graham, B. The Value Added by Electrodiagnostic Testing in the Diagnosis of Carpal Tunnel Syndrome. *J. Bone Jt. Surg.* **2008**, *90*, 2587–2593. [CrossRef]
17. Padua, L.; Lomonaco, M.; Aulisa, L.; Tamburrelli, F.; Valente, E.M.; Padua, R.; Gregori, B.; Tonali, P. Surgical prognosis in carpal tunnel syndrome: Usefulness of a preoperative neurophysiological assessment. *Acta Neurol. Scand.* **1996**, *94*, 343–346. [CrossRef]
18. Sunderland, S.; Smith, J.W. Nerves and nerve injuries. *Plast. Reconstr. Surg.* **1969**, *44*, 601. [CrossRef]
19. Cranford, C.S.; Ho, J.Y.; Kalainov, D.M.; Hartigan, B.J. Carpal Tunnel Syndrome. *J. Am. Acad. Orthop. Surg.* **2007**, *15*, 537–548. [CrossRef]
20. Padua, L.; Coraci, D.; Erra, C.; Pazzaglia, C.; Paolasso, I.; Loreti, C.; Caliandro, P.; Hobson-Webb, L.D. Carpal tunnel syndrome: Clinical features, diagnosis, and management. *Lancet Neurol.* **2016**, *15*, 1273–1284. [CrossRef]
21. Mukaka, M.M. Statistics corner: A guide to appropriate use of correlation coefficient in medical research. *Malawi Med. J.* **2012**, *24*, 69–71.
22. Schober, P.; Boer, C.; Schwarte, L.A. Correlation Coefficients: Appropriate Use and Interpretation. *Anesth. Analg.* **2018**, *126*, 1763–1768. [CrossRef] [PubMed]
23. Di Stefano, V.; Gagliardo, A.; Barbone, F.; Vitale, M.; Ferri, L.; Lupica, A.; Iacono, S.; Di Muzio, A.; Brighina, F. Median-to-Ulnar Nerve Communication in Carpal Tunnel Syndrome: An Electrophysiological Study. *Neurol. Int.* **2021**, *13*, 304–314. [CrossRef] [PubMed]
24. Ise, M.; Saito, T.; Katayama, Y.; Nakahara, R.; Shimamura, Y.; Hamada, M.; Senda, M.; Ozaki, T. Relationship between clinical outcomes and nerve conduction studies before and after surgery in patients with carpal tunnel syndrome. *BMC Musculoskelet. Disord.* **2021**, *22*, 882. [CrossRef] [PubMed]
25. Nanno, M.; Kodera, N.; Tomori, Y.; Hagiwara, Y.; Takai, S. Electrophysiological Assessment for Splinting in the Treatment of Carpal Tunnel Syndrome. *Neurol. Med.-Chir.* **2017**, *57*, 472–480. [CrossRef]
26. Watson, J.C. The Electrodiagnostic Approach to Carpal Tunnel Syndrome. *Neurol. Clin.* **2012**, *30*, 457–478. [CrossRef]
27. Afshar, A.; Tabrizi, A.; Tajbakhsh, M.; Navaeifar, N. Subjective Outcomes of Carpal Tunnel Release in Patients with Diabetes and Patients without Diabetes. *J. Hand Microsurg.* **2019**, *12*, 183–188. [CrossRef]
28. Chen, S.-R.; Ho, T.-Y.; Shen, Y.-P.; Li, T.-Y.; Su, Y.-C.; Lam, K.H.S.; Chen, L.-C.; Wu, Y.-T. Comparison of short- and long-axis nerve hydrodissection for carpal tunnel syndrome: A prospective randomized, single-blind trial. *Int. J. Med. Sci.* **2021**, *18*, 3488–3497. [CrossRef]

29. Martikkala, L.; Mäkelä, K.; Himanen, S.-L. Reduction in median nerve cross-sectional area at the forearm correlates with axon loss in carpal tunnel syndrome. *Clin. Neurophysiol. Pract.* **2021**, *6*, 209–214. [CrossRef]
30. Matesanz, L.; Hausheer, A.C.; Baskozos, G.; Bennett, D.L.; Schmid, A.B. Somatosensory and psychological phenotypes associated with neuropathic pain in entrapment neuropathy. *Pain* **2021**, *162*, 1211–1220. [CrossRef]
31. Moon, H.; Lee, B.J.; Park, D. Change to movement and morphology of the median nerve resulting from steroid injection in patients with mild carpal tunnel syndrome. *Sci. Rep.* **2020**, *10*, 15067. [CrossRef] [PubMed]
32. Sartorio, F.; Negro, F.D.; Bravini, E.; Ferriero, G.; Corna, S.; Invernizzi, M.; Vercelli, S. Relationship between nerve conduction studies and the Functional Dexterity Test in workers with carpal tunnel syndrome. *BMC Musculoskelet. Disord.* **2020**, *21*, 15607. [CrossRef] [PubMed]
33. Sasaki, Y.; Terao, T.; Saito, E.; Ohara, K.; Michishita, S.; Kato, N.; Tani, S.; Murayama, Y. Clinical predictors of surgical outcomes of severe carpal tunnel syndrome patients: Utility of palmar stimulation in a nerve conduction study. *BMC Musculoskelet. Disord.* **2020**, *21*, 725. [CrossRef] [PubMed]
34. Wang, Q.; Chu, H.; Wang, H.; Jin, Y.; Zhao, X.; Weng, C.; Lu, Z. Ring finger sensory latency difference in the diagnosis and treatment of carpal tunnel syndrome. *BMC Neurol.* **2021**, *21*, 432. [CrossRef] [PubMed]

Article

Weight-Related and Personal Risk Factors of Carpal Tunnel Syndrome in the Northern Finland Birth Cohort 1966

Kaisa Lampainen [1,*], Rahman Shiri [2], Juha Auvinen [3,4], Jaro Karppinen [3,5], Jorma Ryhänen [1] and Sina Hulkkonen [1]

1. Department of Hand Surgery, Helsinki University Hospital and University of Helsinki, 00014 Helsinki, Finland; jorma.ryhanen@icloud.com (J.R.); sina.hulkkonen@helsinki.fi (S.H.)
2. Finnish Institute of Occupational Health, 00032 Helsinki, Finland; rahman.shiri@ttl.fi
3. Medical Research Center Oulu, University of Oulu and Oulu University Hospital, 90014 Oulu, Finland; juha.auvinen@oulu.fi (J.A.); jaro.karppinen@oulu.fi (J.K.)
4. Center for Life Course Health Research, University of Oulu, 90014 Oulu, Finland
5. Rehabilitation Services of South Karelia Social and Health Care District, 53130 Lappeenranta, Finland
* Correspondence: kaisa.lampainen@gmail.com

Abstract: Background: Excess body mass is a risk factor for carpal tunnel syndrome (CTS), but the mechanisms of this are unclear. This study aimed to evaluate the association between CTS and personal risk factors of body mass index (BMI), waist circumference and waist-to-hip ratio (WHR). Methods: The study sample consisted of the Northern Finland Birth Cohort 1966 (n = 9246). At the age of 31 in 1997 and at the age of 46 in 2012, the participants underwent a clinical examination. Cohort A consisted of complete cases with a follow-up from 1997 to 2012 (n = 4701), and Cohort B was followed up from 2012 to 2018 (n = 4548). The data on diagnosed CTS were provided by the Care Register for Health Care until the end of 2018. Results: After an adjustment for confounding factors, BMI was associated with CTS among women (hazard ratio (HR) 1.47, 95% Cl 0.98–2.20 for overweight women and HR 2.22, 95% Cl 1.29–3.83 for obese women) and among both sexes combined (HR 1.35 95% Cl 0.96–1.90 for overweight and HR 1.98 95% Cl 1.22–3.22 for obese participants). Neither waist circumference nor WHR was associated with CTS. Conclusions: BMI is an independent risk factor for CTS and is more relevant for estimating the increased risk of CTS due to excess body mass than waist circumference or WHR.

Keywords: carpal tunnel syndrome; body mass index; waist circumference; waist-to-hip ratio; obesity; median nerve

1. Introduction

Carpal tunnel syndrome (CTS) is the most common entrapment neuropathy of the upper extremities and carpal tunnel release is the most common surgical procedure for the upper extremities [1–3]. CTS causes work disability and a great economic burden [4,5]. Based on previous studies, the incidence rate of CTS per 100,000 person-years varies between 88 and 105 among men and 193 and 232 among women, and these rates increase until middle age among both genders [6–8].

Well-known risk factors for CTS are age, female gender, overweight, diabetes mellitus and thyroid disease [7,9–16]. Arthritis, pregnancy and hand trauma are also potential risk factors for CTS [15–17]. The role of smoking as a risk factor for CTS is unclear [18].

Both overweight and obesity are also risk factors, but the mechanism of this is unclear [19]. Only a few case-control and cross-sectional studies have investigated the relationship between waist circumference and CTS [12,20–22] and found an association between the two. In their case-control study, Mondelli and colleagues (2014) showed that a high waist-to-hip (WHR) ratio (>0.95 for men and >0.85 for women) is an independent risk factor for CTS. They found that obese participants (BMI ≥ 30) were at an increased risk of CTS despite their WHR, whereas overweight participants (BMI 25–29.9) were only at risk if their WHR was high [20]. A previous longitudinal study found no association between waist circumference or WHR and carpal tunnel release after controlling for confounding factors [23].

This large birth cohort study aimed to evaluate the association between CTS and personal risk factors, including BMI, waist circumference and WHR.

2. Materials and Methods

2.1. Study Population

The study population consisted of the Northern Finland Birth Cohort 1966 (NFBC1966), which originally consisted of 12,231 participants with an expected date of birth in 1966, born in the Oulu and Lapland provinces [24]. These cohort participants have been studied at several time points throughout their lives. We used data collected in 1997, when they were aged 31 (baseline population, cohort A) and in 2012, when they were 46 (follow-up population, Cohort B) (Figure 1) [25]. When handling the data, we replaced each participant's personal identification number with a study identification code. The study was approved by the Northern Ostrobothnia Hospital District Ethical Committee 94/2011 (12 December 2011), and followed the principles of the Declaration of Helsinki.

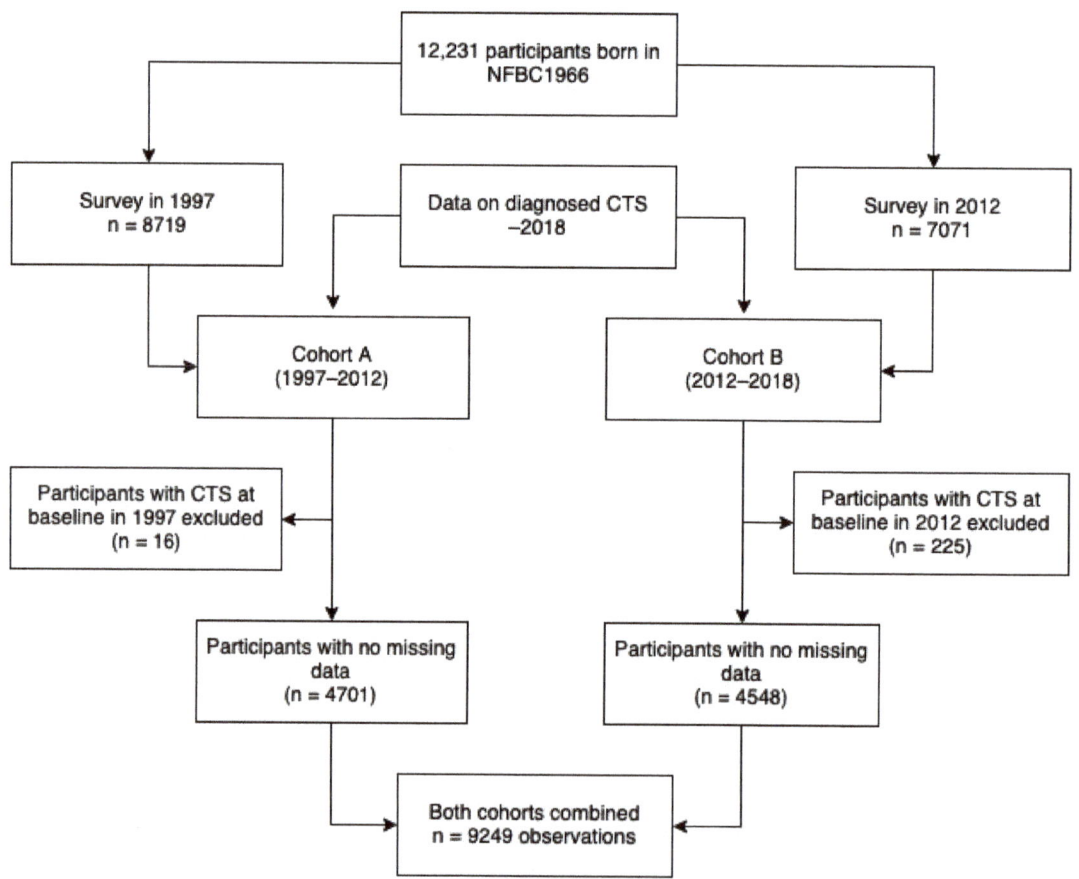

Figure 1. Flowchart of NFBC1966 study population.

2.2. Cohort A (1997–2012)

In 1997, at the age of 31, a total of 8719 participants gave their informed consent to voluntarily participate in the study, underwent a clinical examination, and answered several questionnaires. Of this study population, 16 participants were already diagnosed with CTS and were excluded from the analysis. Of the 8703 participants, 4701 with no missing data were included in the study.

2.3. Cohort B (2012–2018)

The second follow-up study was conducted in 2012 when the cohort was 46 years old. In total, 7071 participants gave their written consent to voluntarily participate in the study, underwent a clinical examination, and answered several questionnaires. Of these, 225 participants were diagnosed with CTS before the second follow-up study and were excluded. Finally, 4548 participants were complete cases and were included in the study.

2.4. Data Collection 1997 and 2012

The participants attended the clinical examination and answered several questionnaires. We measured their weight and height, their waist and hip circumference and calculated their body mass index (BMI) and WHR. BMI, waist circumference and WHR were divided into three categories according to WHO: normal (18.5–24.9 kg/m^2), overweight (25.0–29.9 kg/m^2) and obese (>30 kg/m^2); low risk (<94 cm for men and <80 cm for women), intermediate risk (94–102 cm for men and 80–88 cm for women), and high risk (>102 cm for men and >88 cm for women); low risk ($\leq$0.95 for men and $\leq$0.80 for women), intermediate risk (0.96–1.0 for men and 0.81–0.85 for women), and high risk (>1.0 for men and $\geq$0.86 for women), respectively.

Socio-economic status was defined according to Statistics Finland's Classification of Socio-economic Groups 1989 [26]. This classification divides people into nine categories: farmers, entrepreneurs, upper and lower clerical workers, manual workers, students, pensioners, the unemployed and the unknown. The socio-economic status variable was formed by the following groups: (1) upper clerical workers, (2) lower clerical workers, (3) entrepreneurs, (4) farmers and manual workers (combined), and (5) students, pensioners, and unemployed (combined). If the status was coded as unknown, it was handled as missing data. Information on regular smoking, diabetes, rheumatoid arthritis and thyroid diseases was collected. Cohort A included complete cases and was followed up from 1997 to 2012 (n = 4701), and Cohort B from 2012 to 2018 (n= 4548), forming a total study sample of n = 9249.

2.5. Data on Diagnosed Carpal Tunnel Syndrome

The data on diagnosed CTS were provided by the Care Register for Health Care, which is a national register covering public and private hospital data in Finland. It identifies over 95% of hospital discharges and 80–99% of common diagnoses [27]. It contains information on patients' demographic characteristics, diagnoses, surgical procedures and admission and discharge dates. The diagnoses are coded according to the International Classification of Diagnoses (ICD). According to the eighth revision of ICD 1981–1986, CTS was coded as 357.2; in line with the ninth revision of ICD 1987–1995, as 354.0; and according to the tenth revision in 1996–2016, CTS was coded as G56.0. The diagnoses were obtained from hospital data covering inpatient and outpatient data in specialist care. In specialist care in Finland, the diagnosis of CTS is based on clinical findings and positive electroneuromyography (ENMG) findings.

2.6. Statistical Analyses

The Cox proportional hazards regression model was used to study the association between baseline characteristics and CTS, controlled for panel data. First, we ran sex-specific age-adjusted models or age- and sex-adjusted models for both sexes combined. An association was considered statistically significant if the 95% confidence interval (CI) of the hazard ratio (HR) did not include 1. In these cases, the variables associated with CTS were added to the full models. BMI, waist circumference and WHR were added to the models one at a time. Next, both BMI and waist circumference were added simultaneously to the models. Finally, a multiplicative interaction between BMI (continuous variable) and the other baseline factors was tested.

3. Results

The mean follow-up time was 14.69 (SD 1.66) years for Cohort A, 4.48 (SD 0.41) years for Cohort B and 9.67 (SD 5.25) years for both cohorts combined. A total of 290 participants (3.1%) were diagnosed with CTS during follow-up. The incidence of CTS was higher among women than among men, as, during the follow-up, 4.0% of women and 2.2% of men were diagnosed with CTS. We also found that 51.7% of the study population had increased BMI. In the univariable analysis of both genders combined, overweight and obesity measured by BMI, increased waist circumference, and increased WHR were also associated with CTS (Table 1). The results of the sex-specific analyses for women were similar to those for both genders combined. Among men, obesity and increased waist circumference were associated with CTS (Table 2).

Table 1. Age-adjusted hazard ratios (HR) with 95% confidence intervals (CI) of diagnosed carpal tunnel syndrome among men, women and both genders combined (n = 9249). NA = not applicable.

Characteristic	Women				Men				Both Genders			
	n	Cases	HR	95% CI	n	Cases	HR	95% CI	n	Cases	HR	95% CI
Sex												
Men					4408	96			4408	96		
Women	4841	194							4841	194	1.95	1.47–2.57
Occupational class												
Upper clerical workers	866	16	1		918	3	1		1784	19	1	
Lower clerical workers	1729	66	1.77	1.00–3.12	780	12	4.49	1.27–15.9	2509	78	2.23	1.32–3.76
Entrepreneurs	265	10	2.74	1.20–6.22	397	8	7.22	1.92–27.2	662	18	3.50	1.80–6.79
Farmers, manual workers	1743	92	3.54	2.02–6.20	2139	71	10.09	3.16–32.2	3882	163	4.53	2.76–7.43
students, pensioners, unemployed	238	10	280	1.25–6.27	174	2	3.82	0.64–22.86	412	12	3.03	1.45–6.32
Body mass index												
Normal	2672	84	1		1798	30	1		4470	114	1	
Overweight	1388	61	1.71	1.00–3.12	1965	45	1.53	0.93–2.52	3353	106	1.64	1.24–2.18
Obese	781	49	2.75	1.86–4.06	645	21	2.52	1.32–4.81	1426	70	2.69	1.92–3.75
Waist circumference according to WHO												
Low risk	2213	73	1		2532	46	1		4745	119	1	
Intermediate risk	1052	43	1.57	1.06–2.31	1010	26	1.73	1.05–2.84	2062	69	1.63	1.20–2.21
High risk	1576	78	2.22	1.55–3.17	866	24	2.16	1.20–3.87	2442	102	2.21	1.63–3.00
Waist-hip ratio according to WHO												
Low risk	1417	53	1		1155	23	1		2572	76	1	
Intermediate risk	1210	51	1.56	1.06–2.29	2286	52	1.45	0.89–2.36	3496	103	1.51	1.11–2.04
High risk	2214	90	1.87	1.28–2.75	967	21	1.88	0.96–3.66	3181	111	1.86	1.34–2.60
Regular smoking												
No	2508	73	1		1896	30	1		4404	103	1	
Yes	2333	121	1.90	1.40–2.59	2512	66	1.73	1.07–2.81	4845	187	1.85	1.42–2.40
Diabetes												
No	4731	187	1		4326	93	1		9057	280	1	
Yes	110	7	1.89	0.89–4.00	82	3	2.28	0.70–7.36	192	10	2.01	1.06–3.78
Thyroid disease												
No	4584	186	1		4346	95	1		8930	281	1	
Yes	257	8	0.93	0.46–1.88	62	1	0.86	0.12–6.22	319	9	0.92	0.47–1.77
Rheumatoid arthritis												
No	4767	191	1		4379	95	1		9146	286	1	
Yes	74	3	1.05	0.34–3.27	29	1	1.72	0.24–12.3	103	4	1.16	0.43–3.12

Table 2. Sex-specific and combined sexes' full model hazard ratios (HR) with 95% confidence intervals (CI) of diagnosed carpal tunnel syndrome for body mass index (BMI), waist circumference and waist-hip ratio (WHR).

Characteristic	Women		Men		Both Genders	
	HR	95% CI	HR	95% CI	HR	95% CI
Model 1. Waist-hip ratio according to WHO						
Low risk	1		1		1	
Intermediate risk	1.48	1.00–2.17	1.30	0.80–2.13	1.39	1.03–1.88
High risk	1.68	1.15–2.47	1.58	0.81–3.09	1.60	1.14–2.24
Occupational class						
Upper clerical workers	1		1		1	
Lower clerical workers	1.57	0.89–2.80	4.31	1.21–15.30	2.02	1.19–3.42
Entrepreneurs	2.36	1.04–5.34	6.76	1.79–25.52	3.12	1.61–6.06
Farmers, manual workers	2.94	1.66–5.20	9.09	2.85–28.96	3.84	2.33–6.34
Students, pensioners, unemployed	2.38	1.05–5.38	3.46	0.59–20.40	2.60	1.24–5.46
Regular smoking						
No	1		1		1	
Yes	1.65	1.21–2.26	1.36	0.84–2.22	1.56	1.19–2.03
Diabetes						
No	NA		NA		1	
Yes					1.75	0.92–3.32
Model 2. Waist circumference according to WHO						
Low risk	1		1		1	
Intermediate risk	1.52	1.03–2.24	1.66	1.01–2.73	1.57	1.15–2.13
High risk	2.04	1.42–2.92	1.97	1.10–3.53	1.98	1.46–2.70
Occupational class						
Upper clerical workers	1		1		1	
Lower clerical workers	1.55	0.87–2.76	4.40	1.24–15.61	2.00	1.18–3.39
Entrepreneurs	2.33	1.03–5.28	6.77	1.79–25.56	3.10	1.60–6.02
Farmers, manual workers	2.91	1.65–5.13	9.09	2.85–29.06	3.81	2.32–6.28
Students, pensioners, unemployed	2.32	1.03–5.24	3.39	0.58–19.96	2.55	1.22–5.34
Regular smoking						
No	1		1		1	
Yes	1.65	1.21–2.26	1.37	0.84–2.21	1.56	1.20–2.03
Diabetes						
No	NA		NA		1	
Yes					1.57	0.82–3.01
Model 3. Body mass index						
Normal	1		1		1	
Overweight	1.65	1.17–2.33	1.48	0.90–2.45	1.57	1.18–2.09
Obese	2.48	1.68–3.67	2.21	1.16–4.21	2.35	1.67–3.29
Occupational class						
Upper clerical workers	1		1		1	
Lower clerical workers	1.55	0.87–2.73	4.22	1.19–14.99	1.99	1.17–3.36
Entrepreneurs	2.44	1.08–5.52	6.61	1.75–25.01	3.16	1.63–6.12
Farmers, manual workers	2.85	1.62–5.02	8.90	2.78–28.50	3.75	2.73–6.17
Students, pensioners, unemployed	2.29	1.01–5.17	3.40	0.57–20.19	2.53	1.21–5.31
Regular smoking						
No	1		1		1	
Yes	1.66	1.21–2.26	1.38	0.85–2.24	1.57	1.20–2.04
Diabetes						
No	NA		NA		1	
Yes					1.46	0.76–2.80

In the multivariable analysis, BMI was associated with hospitalization for CTS among women and among both sexes combined (Table 3). The HR was 1.47 (95% CI 0.98–2.20) for overweight women and 2.22 (1.29–3.83) for obese women. The HR was 1.35 (0.96–1.90) for overweight and 1.98 (1.22–3.22) for obesity among both sexes combined. Waist circumference and WHR were not associated with CTS.

Table 3. Sex-specific hazard ratios (HR) with 95% confidence intervals (CI) of diagnosed carpal tunnel syndrome. Full model models for men, women and both genders.

Characteristic	Women		Men		Both Genders	
	HR	95% CI	HR	95% CI	HR	95% CI
Occupational class						
Upper clerical workers	1		1		1	
Lower clerical workers	1.53	0.86–2.73	4.31	1.21–15.35	1.98	1.17–3.37
Entrepreneurs	2.44	1.08–5.52	6.69	1.77–25.29	3.16	1.63–6.13
Farmers, manual workers	2.82	1.59–4.98	9.01	2.81–28.84	3.74	2.26–6.17
Students, pensioners, unemployed	2.27	1.00–5.14	3.42	0.58–20.32	2.53	1.20–5.32
Regular smoking						
No	1		1		1	
Yes	1.66	1.21–2.27	1.38	0.85–2.24	1.57	1.20–2.04
Body mass index						
Normal	1		1		1	
Overweight	1.47	0.98–2.20	1.26	0.67–2.39	1.35	0.96–1.90
Obese	2.22	1.29–3.83	1.70	0.63–4.55	1.98	1.22–3.22
Waist circumference according to WHO						
Low risk	1		1		1	
Intermediate risk	1.22	0.73–2.03	1.51	0.78–2.92	1.35	0.91–1.99
High risk	1.22	0.62–2.41	1.59	0.59–4.33	1.37	0.78–2.40
Waist-hip ratio according to WHO						
Low risk	1		1		1	
Intermediate risk	1.17	0.76–1.81	0.92	0.54–1.56	1.05	0.75–1.48
High risk	0.97	0.53–1.77	0.74	0.34–1.59	0.87	0.54–1.40
Diabetes						
No					1	
Yes					1.50	0.78–2.88

In the multivariable analysis, lower clerical workers, entrepreneurs, farmers and manual workers were at a higher risk of CTS than upper clerical workers among both genders combined, men, and women. After an adjustment for confounding factors, regular smoking was associated with CTS among women and both genders combined. We found no statistically significant association between diabetes, rheumatoid arthritis or thyroid diseases and CTS.

There were no interactions between BMI and gender, between BMI and smoking, between BMI and socio-economic status, between BMI and WHR, or between BMI and waist circumference in terms of risk of CTS.

4. Discussion

Our study showed that excess body mass is an independent risk factor for CTS. However, this association was statistically significant among women and both genders combined. This finding is in line with those of previously published studies. In 2015, Shiri et al. published a meta-analysis of 58 studies, which revealed that excess body mass increased the risk of CTS and that overweight and obesity were associated with CTS in a dose–response relationship [19].

The mechanisms by which excess body mass increases the risk of CTS are not fully understood. Adipose tissue in the carpal tunnel may tighten the tunnel, leading to median nerve compression [28]. Increased pressure in the carpal tunnel may also decrease blood circulation, leading to median nerve ischemia, demyelination and axonal loss [29]. Another possible mechanism is metabolic syndrome causing median nerve injury by adipose deposition, affecting extracellular protein glycation, mitochondrial dysfunction and oxidative stress [30]. Tenosynovitis in carpal tunnel, caused by inflammation through metabolic syndrome, is also a potential mechanism [31].

As mentioned earlier, a few previously published studies have found waist circumference as a marker of central obesity to increase the risk of CTS in [12,20–22]. In the current study, increased waist circumference and WHR were associated with an increased risk of CTS in univariable analysis. However, when we controlled for confounding factors, the associations did not remain statistically significant. As the multivariable analysis of the current study shows, BMI is more relevant than waist circumference and WHR for studying the effect of excess body mass on CTS. It is possible, and even probable, that there is multicollinearity between BMI and waist circumference or WHR. However, including all these variables in the same model (Table 3), it seems that BMI is the strongest of these three to estimate the increased risk of CTS in obesity.

As regards to risk factors for CTS other than those that are weight related, the current study showed that regular smokers, lower clerical workers, entrepreneurs, farmers and manual workers are at a higher risk of CTS than non-smokers or upper clerical workers.

Although previous studies have identified potential risk factors for the development of CTS, the majority of these studies have been cross-sectional. The longitudinal nature of the study better defines the causal relationship. In the current study, the follow-up period was long and the sample size was large. The study population was a representative sample of a single-aged cohort with various socio-economic backgrounds and covered nearly all people born in Northern Finland in 1966. The participation rates in the follow-up studies were also very high. Moreover, the specialized care data on diagnosed CTS that we utilized are reliable and comprehensive, identifying over 95% of hospital discharges and 80–99% of common diagnoses [27].

The current study has some limitations. We used the Care Register for Health Care data from only specialist care. In Finland, the healthcare system is divided into health centers (primary care) and hospitals (specialist care). CTS and suspicion of it are usually coded under the same diagnosis code in primary care. Because of this, we used only hospital data. Thus, using only specialist care data might have excluded patients with mild symptoms and those not willing to visit a hospital. Another limitation of the current study is that the baseline characteristics might have changed over the long follow-up period. Finally, residual confounding may have occurred, and the study did not measure all the risk factors of CTS.

This study showed that BMI is an independent risk factor for CTS and is more relevant than waist circumference or WHR for estimating the effect of excess body mass on the risk of CTS. Future epidemiological studies should investigate whether weight loss as a primary prevention measure decreases the burden of CTS.

Author Contributions: Conceptualization, K.L., S.H., R.S. and J.R.; methodology, S.H. and R.S.; validation, K.L. and S.H.; writing—original draft preparation, K.L.; writing—review and editing, K.L., S.H., R.S. and J.R.; supervision, S.H., R.S., J.A., J.K. and J.R. All authors have read and agreed to the published version of the manuscript.

Funding: Open access funding provided by University of Helsinki. NFBC1966 received financial support from the University of Oulu, Grant no. 65354 and 24000692, Oulu University Hospital, Grant no. 2/97, 8/97 and 24301140, the Ministry of Health and Social Affairs, Grant no. 23/251/97, 160/97, 190/97, the National Institute for Health and Welfare, Helsinki, Grant no. 54121, the Regional Institute of Occupational Health, Oulu, Finland, Grant no. 50621, 54231, the ERDF European Regional Development Fund, Grant no. 539/2010 A31592. This research was funded by a Rehabilitation Foundation Peurunka research grant awarded to K.L., grant number 2021, and the Finnish Medical Foundation grant for S.H., grant number 5302.

Institutional Review Board Statement: The study was conducted in accordance with the Declaration of Helsinki and approved by the Ethics Committee of Northern Ostrobothnia (ETTMK 107/2017).

Informed Consent Statement: Informed consent was obtained from all those involved in the study.

Data Availability Statement: NFBC data is available from the University of Oulu, Infrastructure for Population Studies. Permission to use the data can be applied for research purposes via the electronic material request portal. In the use of data, we follow the EU general data protection regulation (679/2016) and Finnish Data Protection Act. The use of personal data is based on cohort participants' written informed consent at his/her latest follow-up study, which may cause limitations to its use. Please, contact the NFBC project center (NFBCprojectcenter(at)oulu.fi) and visit the cohort website for more information.

Acknowledgments: We thank all cohort members and researchers who participated in the 31 and 47 years studies. We also wish to acknowledge the work of the NFBC project center. We thank Rehabilitation Foundation Peurunka for K.L.'s research grant and the Finnish Medical Foundation for S.H.'s research grant.

Conflicts of Interest: The authors declare no conflict of interest.

References

1. Atroshi, I.; Gummesson, C.; Johnsson, R.; Ornstein, E.; Ranstam, J.; Rosén, I. Prevalence of carpal tunnel syndrome in a general population. *JAMA* **1999**, *282*, 153–158. [CrossRef] [PubMed]
2. de Krom, M.C.; Knipschild, A.D.; Kester, C.T.; Thijs, P.F.; Boekkooi, P.F.; Spaans, F. Carpal tunnel syndrome: Prevalence in the general population. *J. Clin. Epidemiol.* **1992**, *45*, 373–376. [CrossRef]
3. Jain, N.B.; Higgins, L.D.; Losina, E.; Collins, J.; Blazar, P.E.; Katz, J.N. Epidemiology of musculoskeletal upper extremity ambulatory surgery in the United States. *BMC Musculoskelet Disord.* **2014**, *15*, 4. [CrossRef] [PubMed]
4. Feuerstein, M.; Miller, V.L.; Burrell, L.M.; Berger, R. Occupational upper extremity disorders in the federal workforce. Prevalence, health care expenditures, and patterns of work disability. *J. Occup. Environ. Med.* **1998**, *40*, 546–555. [CrossRef] [PubMed]
5. Foley, M.; Silverstein, B.; Polissar, N. The economic burden of carpal tunnel syndrome: Long-term earnings of CTS claimants in Washington State. *Am. J. Ind. Med.* **2007**, *50*, 155–172. [CrossRef] [PubMed]
6. Hulkkonen, S.; Lampainen, K.; Auvinen, J.; Miettunen, J.; Karppinen, J.; Ryhänen, J. Incidence and operations of median, ulnar and radial entrapment neuropathies in Finland: A nationwide register study. *J. Hand Surg. Eur. Vol.* **2020**, *45*, 226–230. [CrossRef] [PubMed]
7. Latinovic, R.; Gulliford, M.C.; Hughes, R.A. Incidence of common compressive neuropathies in primary care. *J. Neurol. Neurosurg. Psychiatry* **2006**, *77*, 263–265. [CrossRef] [PubMed]
8. Tadjerbashi, K.; Åkersson, A.; Atroshi, I. Incidence of referred carpal tunnel syndrome and carpal tunnel release surgery in general population: Increased over the time and reginal variations. *J. Orthop. Surg.* **2019**, *27*, 2309499019825572. [CrossRef] [PubMed]
9. Roquelaure, Y.; Ha, C.; Leclerc, A.; Touranchet, A.; Sauteron, M.; Melchior, M.; Imbernon, E.; Goldberg, M. Epidemiologic surveillance of upper-extremity musculoskeletal disorders in the working population. *Arthritis Rheum.* **2006**, *55*, 765–778. [CrossRef]
10. Mondelli, M.; Giannini, F.; Giacchi, M. Carpal Tunnel Syndrome Incidence in a General Population. *Neurology* **2002**, *58*, 289–294. [CrossRef]
11. Werner, R.A.; Albers, J.W.; Franzblau, A.; Armstrong, T.J. The relationship between body mass index and the diagnosis of carpal tunnel syndrome. *Muscle Nerve* **1994**, *17*, 632–636. [CrossRef] [PubMed]
12. Shiri, R.; Heliövaara, M.; Moilanen, L.; Viikari, J.; Liira, H.; Viikari-Juntura, E. Associations of cardiovascular risk factors, carotid intima-media thickness and manifest atherosclerotic vascular disease with carpal tunnel syndrome. *BMC Musculoskelet. Disord.* **2011**, *12*, 80. [CrossRef] [PubMed]
13. Atroshi, I.; Gummesson, C.; Ornstein, E.; Johnsson, R.; Ranstam, J. Carpal tunnel syndrome and keyboard use at work: A population-based study. *Arthritis Rheum.* **2007**, *56*, 3620–3625. [CrossRef] [PubMed]
14. Musolin, K.; Ramsey, J.G.; Wassell, J.T.; Hard, D.L. Prevalence of carpal tunnel syndrome among employees at a poultry processing plant. *Appl. Ergon.* **2014**, *45*, 1377–1383. [CrossRef] [PubMed]
15. Geoghegan, J.M.; Clark, D.I.; Bainbridge, L.C.; Smith, C.; Hubbard, R. Risk factors in carpal tunnel syndrome. *J. Hand Surg. Br.* **2004**, *29*, 315–320. [CrossRef] [PubMed]
16. Harris-Adamson, C.; Eisen, E.A.; Dale, A.M.; Evanoff, B.; Hegmann, K.T.; Thiese, M.S.; Kapellusch, J.M.; Garg, A.; Burt, S.; Bao, S.; et al. Personal and workplace psychosocial risk factors for carpal tunnel syndrome: A pooled study cohort. *Occup. Environ. Med.* **2013**, *70*, 529–537. [CrossRef] [PubMed]
17. Shiri, R. Arthritis as a risk factor for carpal tunnel syndrome: A meta-analysis. *Scand. J. Rheumatol.* **2016**, *45*, 339–346. [CrossRef] [PubMed]
18. Pourmemari, M.H.; Viikari-Juntura, E.; Shiri, R. Smoking and carpal tunnel syndrome: A meta-analysis. *Muscle Nerve* **2014**, *49*, 345–350. [CrossRef] [PubMed]
19. Shiri, R.; Pourmemari, M.H.; Falah-Hassani, K.; Viikari-Juntura, E. The effect of excess body mass on the risk of carpal tunnel syndrome: A meta-analysis of 58 studies. *Obes. Rev.* **2015**, *16*, 1094–1104. [CrossRef] [PubMed]
20. Mondelli, M.; Aretini, A.; Ginanneschi, F.; Greco, G.; Mattioli, S. Waist circumference and waist-to-hip ratio in carpal tunnel syndrome: A case-control study. *J. Neurol. Sci.* **2014**, *338*, 207–213. [CrossRef] [PubMed]

21. Plastino, M.; Fava, A.; Carmela, C.; De Bartolo, M.; Ermio, C.; Cristiano, D.; Ettore, M.; Abenavoli, L.; Bosco, D. Insulin resistance increases risk of carpal tunnel syndrome: A case-control study. *J. Peripher. Nerv. Syst.* **2011**, *16*, 186–190. [CrossRef] [PubMed]
22. Uzar, E.; Ilhan, A.; Ersoy, A. Association between carpal tunnel syndrome and abdominal obesity. *Turk. J. Neurol.* **2010**, *16*, 187–192.
23. Pourmemari, M.H.; Heliövaara, M.; Viikari-Juntura, E.; Shiri, R. Carpal tunnel release: Lifetime prevalence, annual incidence, and risk factors. *Muscle Nerve* **2018**, *58*, 497–502. [CrossRef] [PubMed]
24. University of Oulu: Northern Finland Birth Cohort 1966. University of Oulu. Available online: http://urn.fi/urn:nbn:fi:att:bc1e5408-980e-4a62-b899-43bec3755243 (accessed on 1 November 2021).
25. Nordström, T.; Miettunen, J.; Auvinen, J.; Ala-Mursula, L.; Keinänen-Kiukaanniemi, S.; Veijola, J.; Järvelin, M.-R.; Sebert, S.; Männikkö, M. Cohort Profile: 46 years of follow-up of the Northern Finland Birth Cohort 1966 (NFBC1966). *Int. J. Epidemiol.* **2022**, *50*, 1786–1787. [CrossRef] [PubMed]
26. Statistics Finland. Classification of Socio-economic Groups 1989. Available online: https://www.stat.fi/en/luokitukset/sosioekon_asema/ (accessed on 1 November 2021).
27. Sund, R. Quality of the Finnish Hospital Discharge Register: A systematic review. *Scand. J. Public Health* **2012**, *40*, 505–515. [CrossRef] [PubMed]
28. Bland, J.D. Carpal tunnel syndrome. *Curr. Opin. Neurol.* **2005**, *18*, 581–585. [CrossRef] [PubMed]
29. Bland, J.D. Carpal tunnel syndrome. *BMJ* **2007**, *335*, 343–346. [CrossRef] [PubMed]
30. Callaghan, B.; Feldman, E. The metabolic syndrome and neuropathy: Therapeutic challenges and opportunities. *Ann. Neurol.* **2013**, *74*, 397–403. [CrossRef] [PubMed]
31. Rechardt, M.; Viikari-Juntura, E.; Shiri, R. Adipokines as predictors of recovery from upper extremity soft tissue disorders. *Rheumatology* **2014**, *53*, 2238–2242. [CrossRef] [PubMed]

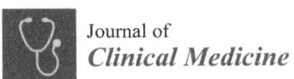

Article

Signs Indicative of Central Sensitization Are Present but Not Associated with the Central Sensitization Inventory in Patients with Focal Nerve Injury

Luis Matesanz-García [1,2], Ferran Cuenca-Martínez [3], Ana Isabel Simón [4], David Cecilia [5,6,7], Carlos Goicoechea-García [8,9], Josué Fernández-Carnero [9,10,*,†] and Annina B. Schmid [11,*,†]

1. Escuela Internacional de Doctorado, Department of Physical Therapy, Occupational Therapy, Rehabilitation and Physical Medicine, Rey Juan Carlos University, 28922 Alcorcón, Spain; luis.matesanzgarcia@gmail.com
2. Department of Physiotherap, Centro Superior de Estudios Universitarios La Salle, Universidad Autónoma de Madrid, 28023 Madrid, Spain
3. Exercise Intervention for Health Research Group (EXINH-RG), Department of Physiotherapy, University of Valencia, 46010 Valencia, Spain; fecuen2@gmail.com
4. Unit of Elbow-Hand, Service de Traumatología, Hospital Severo Ochoa, 28911 Leganés, Spain; ai.simoncarrascal@gmail.com
5. Unit of Elbow-Hand, Service de Traumatología, Hospital 12 de Octubre, 28048 Madrid, Spain; dacecilia@hotmail.com
6. Complutense University of Madrid, 28040 Madrid, Spain
7. Department of Surgery, Hospital Vithas La Milagrosa, 28010 Madrid, Spain
8. Department Basic Health Sciences, Rey Juan Carlos University, 28922 Alcorcón, Spain; carlos.goicoechea@urjc.es
9. Grupo Multidisciplinar de Investigación y Tratamiento del Dolor, Grupo de Excelencia Investigadora URJC-Banco de Santander, 28922 Madrid, Spain
10. Department of Physical Therapy, Occupational Therapy, Rehabilitation and Physical Medicine, Rey Juan Carlos University, 28922 Alcorcón, Spain
11. Nuffield Department of Clinical Neurosciences, University of Oxford, Oxford OX3 9DU, UK
* Correspondence: josue.fernandez@urjc.es (J.F.-C.); annina.schmid@neuro-research.ch (A.B.S.)
† These authors contributed equally to this work.

Abstract: Objective: Carpal tunnel syndrome (CTS) is the most common focal nerve injury. People with CTS may show alterations in central processing of nociceptive information. It remains unclear whether the central sensitization inventory (CSI) is capable of detecting such altered central pain processing. Methods: Thirty healthy volunteers were matched with 30 people with unilateral CTS from the orthopaedic waitlist. Changes to central pain processing were established through psychophysical sensory testing (bilateral pressure pain thresholds (PPT), conditioned pain modulation, temporal summation) and pain distribution on body charts. Patients also completed pain severity and function questionnaires, psychological questionnaires and the CSI. Results: Compared to healthy volunteers, patients with CTS have lower PPTs over the carpal tunnel bilaterally (t = −4.06, $p < 0.0001$ ipsilateral and t = −4.58, $p < 0.0001$ contralateral) and reduced conditioned pain modulation efficacy (t = −7.31, $p < 0.0001$) but no differences in temporal summation (t = 0.52, $p = 0.60$). The CSI was not associated with psychophysical measures or pain distributions indicative of altered central pain processing. However, there was a correlation of the CSI with the Beck Depression Inventory (r = 0.426; $p = 0.019$). Conclusion: Patients with CTS show signs of altered central pain mechanisms. The CSI seems unsuitable to detect changes in central pain processing but is rather associated with psychological factors in people with focal nerve injuries.

Keywords: entrapment neuropathy; conditioned pain modulation; temporal summation; pain measurement; carpal tunnel syndrome; pressure pain threshold; central sensitization; central sensitization inventory

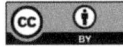

1. Introduction

Carpal tunnel syndrome (CTS) is the most common focal nerve injury [1,2]. It is defined as a compression of the median nerve as it passes through the carpal tunnel in the wrist. Classically, CTS symptoms manifest themselves in the median nerve area, although extramedian or proximal spread of symptoms is frequently reported [3]. This spread of symptoms has been attributed to changes in the central nervous system such as central sensitization [4].

Central sensitization is a neurophysiological mechanism that cannot be directly determined in humans. However, in addition to the spread of symptoms, psychophysical sensory testing can be used to infer the contribution of central pain mechanisms to patients' presentations. For instance, local and remote mechanical hyperalgesia such as measured with pain thresholds has been associated with central sensitization [5,6]. Additionally, temporal summation is related to activity-dependent plasticity within the central nervous system [7,8]. Several studies have examined the presence of such local and widespread hyperalgesia in patients with CTS with conflicting results [9,10].

In addition to increased facilitation, a disruption of inhibitory mechanisms is another central mechanism that can lead to hyperexcitability. Conditioned pain modulation (CPM) is a psychophysical measure that examines the efficacy of endogenous inhibitory systems [11]. CPM evaluates whether a painful test stimulus can be modulated by a noxious conditioning stimulus applied at a remote part of the body. About 70% of patients with chronic pain show signs of reduced CPM efficacy [12]. To date, only one publication has examined possible alterations of the descending inhibitory system by means of CPM in patients with CTS and found reduced efficacy [13].

Whereas these psychophysical sensory tests can provide information about the potential involvement of central pain mechanisms, they are time consuming and involve costly equipment. Thus, self-completed questionnaires have been developed to identify the presence of "central sensitization". For instance, the central sensitization inventory (CSI) has been suggested to identify patients with "central sensitivity syndrome" such as fibromyalgia, chronic fatigue syndrome, irritable bowel or temporomandibular joint disorders [14]. In addition, the CSI is associated with outcomes after spinal surgery [15]. However, recent studies question its construct validity. The CSI was originally validated by demonstrating increasing CSI scores in conditions thought to represent increasing degrees of central sensitization (e.g., healthy controls, regional chronic low back pain, chronic widespread pain, fibromyalgia) [14]. Similarly, the cutoff to identify "central sensitivity syndrome" was determined by receiver operating curve analyses, best distinguishing patients with diagnoses that are thought to be characterised by central mechanisms (e.g., fibromyalgia) from healthy controls [16]. Arguably, a more compelling way of evaluating the construct validity of a tool that is meant to identify central sensitisation is to examine its associations with psychophysical testing. However, recent studies in patients with temporomandibular disorders, shoulder pain, chronic whiplash and chronic spinal pain found no relationship between the CSI and psychophysical tests indicating the presence of central pain mechanisms [17–20]. In contrast, other studies have identified a weak correlation of the CSI with mechanical hyperalgesia and CPM in patients with knee osteoarthritis [21], and CSI scores seem higher in patients with musculoskeletal pain and more impaired CPM [22]. Of note, evidence is growing that the CSI is more strongly associated with psychological measures rather than psychophysical measures indicating central pain mechanisms [18–21,23]. To date, construct validity of the CSI has only been evaluated in populations with musculoskeletal pain. It remains unclear how the CSI performs in patients with peripheral nerve injuries.

To improve our knowledge of alterations in pain processing in focal nerve injuries and the construct validity of the CSI, this study has the following objectives: (1) Identify alterations in central pain mechanisms in patients with CTS using psychophysical sensory testing and pain mapping. (2) Investigate whether the CSI is associated with psychophysical parameters and pain distributions indicative of central pain mechanisms. (3) Investigate whether the CSI is associated with psychological parameters.

2. Materials and Methods

2.1. Participants

Thirty patients with unilateral CTS were recruited from Hand and Elbow surgery units from 12 Octubre Hospital and Severo Ochoa Hospital, both located in Madrid. All patients were on the orthopaedic surgery waitlist, with at least one year of persistency of symptoms, had positive Tinel's and Phalen's sign and had electrodiagnostic confirmation of moderate to severe CTS on the affected side according to the American Association of Neuromuscular and Electrodiagnostic Medicine [24]. Patients were excluded if the electrodiagnostic testing identified sensory and/or motor deficits of the radial and/or ulnar nerve, if any indication for nerve root involvement was present (e.g., needle EMG) or if patients reported previous hand surgeries, previous steroid infiltrations, wrist fractures, diagnoses related to the cervical spine and upper limb (e.g., cervical radiculopathies, shoulder injuries), or other musculoskeletal comorbidities (e.g., rheumatoid arthritis and fibromyalgia). Women who were pregnant were excluded from the study.

The patients were matched for age and sex with healthy controls (HC, n = 30). Those were recruited through advertisements around the hospitals and university and through relatives of participating patients. All participants gave informed written consent prior to participating, and the study received ethical clearance from the two committees of the participating hospitals CPMP/ICH/135/95 (Severo Ochoa Hospital, December 2017) and 20/092 (12 Octubre Hospital, March 2020).

2.2. Symptom Characteristics and Functional Deficits

The Boston carpal tunnel questionnaire was used to assess symptom severity and functional deficits. The Boston carpal tunnel questionnaire consists of a symptom and a function subscale [25]. This questionnaire has been validated in Spanish, with good levels of internal consistency and reproducibility [26]. The current hand pain intensity was recorded using a visual analogue scale (VAS), with 0 being no pain and 100 being the worst pain imaginable.

The presence of neuropathic pain was assessed with the Spanish version of Douleur Neuropathique 4 (DN4). This version has shown good internal consistency [27]. The questionnaire consists of an initial part with questions that evaluate a series of neuropathic symptom descriptors (burning and cold-like pain, electric shock, tingling, pins and needles, numbness, itching) followed by a short sensory clinical examination (hypoesthesia to touch, hypoesthesia to pin prick and brush allodynia). A DN4 score of ≥ 4 was interpreted as neuropathic pain [28] and a score < 4 was interpreted as nociceptive pain.

The central sensitization inventory (CSI) is a tool originally designed to identify patients with "central sensitivity syndrome" [14]. It includes a wide range of 25 questions covering pain and stiffness, daily function, psychological factors (e.g., anxiety, depression), fatigue and memory. The Spanish translation shows good reliability and internal consistency [29]. The patient scores each question from 0 to 4: never, rarely, sometimes, continuously and always. The total score ranges from 0 to 100 with values over 40 thought to indicate the presence of "central sensitivity syndrome" [14].

2.3. Signs Indicative of Altered Central Pain Processing

2.3.1. Pressure Pain Threshold (PPT)

PPT is defined as the minimum amount of pressure needed to elicit pain. Measurements of PPT were made using a digital algometer (Model FDX 10®, Wagner Instruments, Greenwich, CT, USA). This instrument measures the pressure in kg/cm^2. The measurements were made bilaterally (affected and unaffected side) over the carpal tunnel (Supplementary Figure S1). The average of three measurements was recorded, with an interval of 30 s between each measurement to avoid a temporal summation effect. PPT has shown good reliability and internal consistency [30].

2.3.2. CPM

For the evaluation of CPM efficiency, an average of three PPT measures was used as a test stimulus over the base of the dorsal side of the distal phalanx of the thumb of the affected side (Supplementary Figure S1). The conditioning stimulus involved ischemic pain using a sphygmomanometer applied on the unaffected arm with a pressure of 200 mmHg until the subjects reported pain intensity between 5–7/10 on a numerical pain rating scale. While the sphygmomanometer was still inflated, the PPT measurements were repeated on the dorsal side of the distal phalanx of the thumb on the affected side. This protocol has been shown to be adequate to assess the endogenous inhibitory system in patients with knee osteoarthritis [31]. CPM efficacy was calculated by deducting the PPT after applying the conditioning stimulus from the PPT obtained before the conditioning stimulus. Positive values indicate effective pain modulation [32].

2.3.3. Temporal Summation

The measurement of temporal summation was performed using a Model FDX 10® digital algometer, Wagner Instruments, Greenwich, CT, USA applied to the intensity of the PPT at the midpoint between the nail and the interphalangeal joint on the dorsal side of the distal phalanx of the first finger of the affected side (Supplementary Figure S1). Numerical pain ratings from 0–10 were obtained for a single stimulus followed by a rating after 10 stimuli with a repetition rate of 1 Hz. For the isolated stimuli, the patients were asked to indicate the onset of pain and rate it from 0–10. The repetitive stimuli were performed in an area around the same point of the finger with the same pressure that induced the first onset of pain during the isolated stimulus. The average pain intensity after 10 repetitions was recorded. The temporal summation ratio was calculated by dividing the average pain produced by the train of stimuli by the pain produced by the single stimulus. A similar method has been used and validated previously [33].

2.3.4. Symptom Spread

Patients marked the localization of symptoms on a hand and body diagram [34]. Results were dichotomized into median and extramedian distribution.

2.4. Emotional Wellbeing

To evaluate emotional wellbeing, patients completed the Beck Depression Inventory (BECK) and the State-Trait Anxiety Inventory (STAI). The BECK consists of 21 elements related to depressive symptoms (e.g., hopelessness and irritability), specific thoughts (e.g., guilt or feelings of being punished) and physical symptoms [35,36]. STAI has demonstrated acceptable psychometric properties in its Spanish version [37].

To assess pain-related fear of movement, the validated Tampa kinesiophobia scale (TSK) was used. Each item is rated on a four-point Likert scale ranging from "strongly agree" to "strongly disagree" with a cutoff of 29 points. This questionnaire has shown a good consistency [38,39].

2.5. Statistical Analyses

The sample size was estimated using the program G*Power 3.1.7 (G*power from University of Dusseldorf, Germany) [40]. The sample size calculation was powered to detect between-group differences in PPT measures. Using previously published data measured over the carpal tunnel area in healthy controls and patients with CTS [41], n = 30 participants are required in each group to detect an effect size of 0.74 with 80% statistical power (alpha = 0.05, independent t-test). This sample size is sufficient to detect large effects in correlation analyses (rho = 0.44, power 80%, alpha 0.05).

We performed the data analysis using the Statistics Package for Social Science (SPSS 20.00, IBM Inc., Armonk, NY, USA). We checked data normality by visual inspection of histograms and the Kolmogorov–Smirnov test. Participants' sociodemographic and clinical characteristics were summarized using descriptive statistics and summary tables.

To determine the presence of signs indicative of altered central pain processing, we employed independent Student's *t*-tests to identify differences between healthy and patient groups for psychophysical variables. The frequency of extraterritorial spread of symptoms (median/extramedian) was reported.

To identify associations between CSI and psychophysical signs indicative of altered pain processing, we performed Pearson's correlation statistics in patient data only. Coefficients of 0.5 or above were interpreted as a strong correlation, 0.3 moderate and 0.1 small correlation. We corrected for false discovery rate using the Benjamini–Hochberg correction (FDR = 25%). We also grouped patients with CTS into those with CSI $\geq$ 40 and <40 and explored differences in psychophysical tests and symptom spread with independent *t*-tests and Chi squared or Fisher's exact test statistics as appropriate.

To explore the relationship between CSI and emotional wellbeing (BECK, TSK, STAI) in patient data, we calculated Pearson correlations coefficients and used Benjamini–Hochberg correction to correct for a false discovery rate. Unadjusted *p*-values are reported for ease of interpretation.

3. Results

Thirty participants were healthy controls (8 men and 22 women with a mean age of 46.23 $\pm$ 1.36 years), and 30 patients diagnosed with CTS (8 men and 22 women with a mean age of 48.67 $\pm$ 1.19 years, Table 1). According to the Boston questionnaire, patients had on average mild to moderate symptoms and moderate to severe function deficits. The mean pain intensity was 4.2/10 (SD 2.7). Using the DN4 questionnaire, the most common pain descriptor was tingling (100%), followed by numbness (96.6%) and electric shocks (90%). In contrast, hypoesthesia to touch and pinprick was present only in 50% and 60% of patients, respectively. Twenty-eight patients (93.3%) were classified as having neuropathic pain according to the DN4.

Table 1. Participant characteristics.

	Healthy (n = 30)	CTS (n = 30)
Female, n (%)	22 (77.3)	22 (77.3)
Age (Years)	46.2 $\pm$ 1.36	48.7 $\pm$ 1.2

Boston
    Severity
    Functional deficits
		2.6 $\pm$ 0.11
		3.5 $\pm$ 0.11

Visual Analogue Scale		4.2 (2.7)
DN4 total score		5.9 (1.6)
Burning, n (%)		11 (36.6)
Painful cold, n (%)		9 (30.0)
Electric shocks, n (%)		27 (90.0)
Tingling, n (%)		30 (100.0)
Pins and needles, n (%)		22 (73.3)
Numbness, n (%)		29 (96.6)
Itching, n (%)		9 (30.0)
Hypoesthesia to touch, n (%)		15 (50.0)
Hypoesthesia to pinprick, n (%)		18 (60.0)
DN4 neuropathic, n (%)		28 (93.3)

Data are shown as mean and standard deviation or n (%).

3.1. Patients with CTS Have Signs Indicative of Altered Central Pain Processing

There were statistically significant differences between patients with CTS and healthy participants in the psychophysical variables related to central pain processing. PPTs were reduced in patients with CTS, indicative of mechanical hyperalgesia compared to healthy controls both on the ipsilateral (t = −4.06; $p < 0.0001$) and contralateral side (t = −4.58; $p < 0.0001$).

Similarly, CPM efficiency was reduced in patients with CTS compared to healthy controls (t = −7.31; $p < 0.01$). No differences were found for temporal summation (t = 0.52, $p = 0.60$). Data are shown in Table 2.

Table 2. Variables indicative of changes in central pain processing.

	Healthy (n = 30)	CTS (n = 30)	*p*-Value
PPT affected side (Kg/cm²)	5.9 (2.0)	3.4 (1.7)	$p < 0.0001$
PPT contralateral side (Kg/cm²)	5.9 (2.0)	3.8 (2.0)	$p < 0.0001$
CPM	2.1 (2.0)	0.1 (0.9)	$p < 0.0001$
Temporal summation ratio	1.5 (0.9)	1.6 (0.9)	$p = 0.60$

Data are shown as mean (standard deviation); PPT: pressure pain threshold; CPM: conditioned pain modulation; *p*-values reflect Student's *t*-tests.

3.2. Association between Central Sensitization Inventory and Signs of Altered Central Pain Processing

The mean CSI in patients with CTS was 32.4 (SD 11.8). Eight patients (26.67%) had a score ≥ 40.

The CSI did not correlate with any psychophysical signs of altered pain processing (Table 3). Similarly, there were no differences in psychophysical signs of altered pain processing if patients were grouped according to the CSI cutoff of ≥40 ($p > 0.600$).

Table 3. Correlations between CSI and signs of altered central pain processing in patients with CTS.

	Pearson Correlation Coefficient	Unadj *p*-Value
CSI vs. PPT affected side	0.023	0.903
CSI vs. PPT unaffected side	−0.042	0.828
CSI vs. CPM	0.276	0.140
CSI vs. temporal summation	0.069	0.719

CSI: central sensitization inventory; PPT: pain pressure threshold; CPM: conditioned pain modulation.

Extramedian distribution of symptoms was reported by 25 (83%) of patients with the remaining patients reporting a median distribution. No difference was identified for the proportion of patients with median/extramedian spread of symptoms according to the CSI cutoff (Table 4).

Table 4. Association between CSI and symptom spread.

CSI	Median	Extramedian	*p*-Value
≥40	1	8	0.521
<40	4	17	

p-values reflect Fisher exact test. CSI: central sensitization inventory.

3.3. Association between Central Sensitization Inventory and Emotional Wellbeing

The mean BECK, STAI and TSK scores in patients with CTS were 7.87 (SD 4.91), 24.30 (SD 5.05), and 25.93 (SD 7.62), respectively (Supplementary Table S1). The CSI did not correlate with the level of anxiety according to STAI (r = 0.026; $p = 0.893$) and kinesiophobia according to TSK (r = 0.109; $p = 0.566$). There was, however, a moderate correlation between CSI and depression according to BECK (r = 0.426; $p = 0.019$, Table 5), which survived the Benjamini–Hochberg correction.

Table 5. Correlations between CSI and emotional wellbeing.

	CTS	
	Pearson Correlation Coefficient	Unadj p-Value
CSI with BECK	0.426	0.019 *
CSI with STAI	0.026	0.893
CSI with TSK	0.109	0.566

* reflects p-value that remains significant after Benjamini–Hochberg correction.

4. Discussion

Our cohort of patients with CTS has clear indications for the presence of central pain mechanisms as apparent by local and widespread mechanical hyperalgesia and impaired CPM compared to healthy volunteers. No changes were apparent for temporal summation. Of note, there was no association of the CSI with psychophysical measures or symptom spread indicative of central pain mechanisms. There was, however, a moderate correlation between the CSI and depression scores, suggesting that the CSI may be more closely related to psychological parameters than psychophysical measures indicative of central pain mechanisms in patients with focal nerve injury.

Our cohort of patients with CTS had clear indication of a presence of central pain mechanisms, although there was heterogeneity among patients. We identified mechanical hyperalgesia both locally as well as remotely, extraterritorial spread of symptoms and lower efficacy of CPM. Extraterritorial spread of symptoms in patients with CTS is consistently reported in the literature [4,42,43] and has been associated with the presence of central mechanisms. Mechanical hyperalgesia is also commonly interpreted as a sign of central sensitization [44,45]. Local (and remote) mechanical hyperalgesia has previously been reported in focal peripheral neuropathies including CTS [9,43,46]. However other patient cohorts could not confirm this at group level [47,48]. This discrepancy may be attributed to different recruitment pathways as well as different sites of PPT measurements (e.g., palmar aspect of index finger, carpal tunnel). Importantly, the large variation in mechanical hyperalgesia within patients with CTS suggests differing extents of central contributions in individual patients.

Intriguingly, this is the second study demonstrating impaired CPM efficacy in patients with CTS (see also Soon et al., 2017) [13]. On the other hand, temporal summation, which is related to activity-dependent plasticity within the central nervous system [7,8] remained unaltered in patients with CTS. Whereas we assessed temporal summation with PPTs as used in other cohorts [33], more established protocols using pinprick stimulators also did not find group differences between patients with CTS and healthy participants [47]. In line with our results, temporal summation is often found to be comparable at group level in other peripheral neuropathies including systemic polyneuropathies [49,50] and other focal nerve injuries [46,51]. Again though, there is variation within patients, suggesting that some patients have elevated temporal summation, which may be washed out in group comparisons.

Of note, we did not identify an association between the CSI and psychophysical measures and symptom location indicative of altered central pain processing. The CSI was originally developed as a tool to identify central sensitization characteristics [52]. It was developed in patients with fibromyalgia, chronic widespread pain and chronic low back pain, who presumably have stronger clinical phenotypes than the here studied patients with entrapment neuropathies. Some studies in musculoskeletal pain report a correlation between the CSI and the spread of pain [21,53]. However, similar to our findings in patients with peripheral nerve injury, other studies do not find a correlation of the CSI with symptom spread in people with shoulder pain [20] and whiplash injury [18], questioning its construct validity.

A recent systematic review reports a high construct validity of the CSI [54]. However, the included studies compared the CSI to other questionnaires related to pain severity, general health, emotional wellbeing or sleep. There may be a reciprocal relationship of these measures with central pain mechanisms. However, these constructs are not measures of central sensitisation, which the CSI is meant to evaluate. Surprisingly, not even the original development of the CSI involved psychophysical measures of central pain mechanisms, which are considered to be best practice when assessing the manifestation of central sensitisation in humans [55]. Recent studies have compared the CSI with psychophysical tests indicative of central pain mechanisms. Of note, most studies find no [17–19] or only a weak correlation [21,53] between the CSI and psychophysical tests in patients with musculoskeletal pain. This, together with our findings of no association between the CSI and psychophysical tests in patients with focal nerve injury, further questions the validity of the CSI in detecting human correlates of central sensitization.

Intriguingly though, the CSI was associated with depressive symptoms determined on the BECK in our cohort. Such an association of CSI with psychological wellbeing has been consistently reported in the literature [17–21,23]. This may not be surprising as several questions of the CSI explore psychological constructs such as anxiety, feeling sad or depressed. Whereas, indeed, a decrease in emotional wellbeing is frequently associated with chronic pain including neuropathic pain [46,49,50,56–58], care has to be taken to not confuse changes in emotional wellbeing with the presence of central sensitisation [59]. Unfortunately, these two distinct principles are often equated in the clinical literature. We should note though that whereas psychological parameters were more pronounced in patients with CTS compared to healthy volunteers in our study, average scores were not considered clinically relevant. These findings are in line with previous reports in patients with CTS [42].

4.1. Limitations

Some limitations have to be taken into account. The sample size was calculated to detect differences in central pain processing between healthy people and patients with CTS. Whereas it was adequately powered to detect large effects on correlations between the CSI and psychophysical testing, small or moderate correlations would have been missed. Inspection of the data, however, clearly demonstrated the absence of trends, and even if larger samples may have detected significant correlations, these would likely have been weak.

We recruited patients from surgery waiting lists, which is likely to include more severe profiles. However, symptom and function severity in our study was comparable with previous CTS cohorts from primary care [60] and secondary care [42]. The examiner who performed psychophysical testing could not be blinded to group allocation (CTS vs. healthy). To minimise bias, the examiner was not aware of the outcome of the CSI and other questionnaires until after psychophysical testing was performed. As per routine practice in participating hospitals, the electrodiagnostic test was only performed on the affected side. Subclinical cases of CTS on the contralateral side may therefore have been missed [61].

4.2. Clinical Implications

Our study confirms the presence of central pain mechanisms in patients with focal nerve injury. This is of clinical relevance as their presence may be associated with poorer prognosis in some musculoskeletal conditions [62]. It has also been suggested that the identification of central pain mechanisms may help personalise management strategies [63], an area of active research. For instance, duloxetine may be particularly effective in patients with peripheral diabetic neuropathy who have altered CPM efficacy [64]. Similarly, CPM efficacy may predict the analgesic effect of non-steroidal antirheumatic inflammatory drugs plus acetaminophen in patients with knee osteoarthritis [65], and temporal summation seems to predict pain relief from ketamine in patients with neuropathic pain [66]. Future studies will have to examine whether the identification of central pain mechanisms may be important not only for pharmacological management but also beyond (e.g., physiotherapy).

Most studies of personalised management according to central pain mechanisms use time-consuming psychophysical testing. A low-cost self-reported questionnaire that identifies central sensitisation as measured by psychophysical tools would be ideal. Unfortunately, our study adds to the increasing body of evidence that questions the usefulness of the CSI in identifying central sensitisation according to psychophysical measures. Rather, our data, together with other studies, consistently suggest that the CSI better reflects emotional wellbeing. It is crucial that the distinct concept of emotional wellbeing is not conflated with the neurophysiological concept of central sensitisation in clinical practice. Nevertheless, even though the CSI may not be detecting "central sensitisation" in a strict sense, it may still be of value clinically. For instance, CSI scores seem to be associated with prognostic outcome in certain musculoskeletal conditions [67,68], and this could be further explored in focal nerve injuries.

5. Conclusions

Our results suggest that patients with CTS have changes indicative of altered central pain processing. The CSI does not seem to be associated with psychophysical measures of central sensitization. Rather, the CSI correlates with emotional wellbeing, in particular, depression scores. These data question the construct validity of the CSI in detecting central sensitisation in patients with focal peripheral nerve injury.

Supplementary Materials: The following supporting information can be downloaded at https://www.mdpi.com/article/10.3390/jcm11041075/s1, Figure S1: Three psychophysical measurements. Table S1: Results of emotional wellbeing questionnaires.

Author Contributions: Conceptualization, L.M.-G., J.F.-C. and C.G.-G.; methodology, L.M.-G., J.F.-C., A.B.S. and F.C.-M.; software J.F.-C.; formal analysis, J.F.-C. and L.M.-G.; investigation, L.M.-G., D.C. and A.I.S.; resources, J.F.-C.; data curation, J.F.-C. and L.M.-G.; writing—original draft preparation, L.M.-G., J.F.-C. and F.C.-M.; writing—review and editing, L.M.-G., J.F.-C., C.G.-G., F.C.-M. and A.B.S.; visualization, J.F.-C.; supervision, J.F.-C., D.C., A.I.S., C.G.-G. and A.B.S. All authors have read and agreed to the published version of the manuscript.

Funding: A.B.S. is supported by a Wellcome Trust Clinical Career Development Fellowship (222101/Z/20/Z). Her research was supported by the National Institute for Health Research (NIHR) Oxford Biomedical Research Centre (BRC). The views expressed are those of the authors and not necessarily those of the NHS, the NIHR or the Department of Health.

Institutional Review Board Statement: The study was conducted in accordance with the Declaration of Helsinki, and approved by the Institutional Review Board (or Ethics Committee) of hospitals CPMP/ICH/135/95 (Severo Ochoa Hospital, December 2017 and 20/092 (12 Octubre Hospital, March 2020).

Informed Consent Statement: Informed consent was obtained from all subjects involved in the study. Written informed consent has been obtained from the participant(s) to publish this paper.

Data Availability Statement: The data presented in this study are available on request from the corresponding author.

Acknowledgments: The authors thank all patients and healthy volunteers for their participation. We would also like to thank both departments of Elbow and Hand surgery units of Severo Ochoa and 12 Octubre Hospitals for their collaboration on the recruitment. Finally, we would like to thank Laura Flix for her help with the assessments.

Conflicts of Interest: The authors declare no conflict of interest.

References

1. Singh, R.; Gamble, G.; Cundy, T. Lifetime risk of symptomatic carpal tunnel syndrome in Type 1 diabetes. *Diabet. Med.* **2005**, *22*, 625–630. [CrossRef] [PubMed]
2. Jenkins, P.J.; Watts, A.C.; Duckworth, A.D.; McEachan, J.E. Socioeconomic deprivation and the epidemiology of carpal tunnel syndrome. *J. Hand Surg. Eur. Vol.* **2012**, *37*, 123–129. [CrossRef] [PubMed]
3. Nora, D.B.; Becker, J.; Ehlers, J.A.; Gomes, I. What symptoms are truly caused by median nerve compression in carpal tunnel syndrome? *Clin. Neurophysiol.* **2005**, *116*, 275–283. [CrossRef] [PubMed]

4. Zanette, G.; Marani, S.; Tamburin, S. Extra-median spread of sensory symptoms in carpal tunnel syndrome suggests the presence of pain-related mechanisms. *Pain* **2006**, *122*, 264–270. [CrossRef]
5. Sorkin, L.S.; Willis, W.D. Neurogenic Hyperalgesia: Central Neural Correlates in Responses of Spinothalamic Tract Neurons. *J. Neurophysiol.* **1991**, *66*, 228–246.
6. Treede, R.D.; Meyer, R.A.; Raja, S.N.; Campbell, J.N. Peripheral and Central Mechanisms of cutaneous hyperalgesia. *Prog. Neurobiol.* **1992**, *38*, 397–421. [CrossRef]
7. Arendt-Nielsen, L.; Brennum, J.; Sindrup, S.; Bak, P. Electrophysiological and psychophysical quantification of temporal summation in the human nociceptive system. *Eur. J. Appl. Physiol. Occup. Physiol.* **1994**, *68*, 266–273. [CrossRef]
8. Koltzenburg, M.; Handwerker, H.O. Differential ability of human cutaneous nociceptors to signal mechanical pain and to produce vasodilatation. *J. Neurosci.* **1994**, *14*, 1756–1765. [CrossRef]
9. Fernandez-De-Las-Peñas, C.; De La Llave-Rincn, A.I.; Fernndez-Carnero, J.; Cuadrado, M.L.; Arendt-Nielsen, L.; Pareja, J.A. Bilateral widespread mechanical pain sensitivity in carpal tunnel syndrome: Evidence of central processing in unilateral neuropathy. *Brain* **2009**, *132*, 1472–1479. [CrossRef]
10. Schmid, A.B.; Soon, B.T.; Wasner, G.; Coppieters, M.W. Can widespread hypersensitivity in carpal tunnel syndrome be substantiated if neck and arm pain are absent? *Eur. J. Pain* **2012**, *16*, 217–228. [CrossRef]
11. Nir, R.; Yarnitsky, D. Conditioned pain modulation. *Curr. Opin. Support. Palliat. Care* **2015**, *9*, 131–137. [CrossRef]
12. Lewis, G.N.; Rice, D.A.; McNair, P.J. Conditioned pain modulation in populations with chronic pain: A systematic review and meta-analysis. *J. Pain* **2012**, *13*, 936–944. [CrossRef]
13. Soon, B.; Vicenzino, B.; Schmid, A.B.; Coppieters, M.W. Facilitatory and inhibitory pain mechanisms are altered in patients with carpal tunnel syndrome. *PLoS ONE* **2017**, *12*, e0183252. [CrossRef]
14. Moser, A.; Range, K.; York, D. The Development and Psychometric Validation of the Central Sensitization Inventory (CSI). *Pain Pract.* **2012**, *12*, 276–285. [CrossRef]
15. Bennett, E.E.; Walsh, K.M.; Thompson, N.R.; Ajit, A. Central Sensitization Inventory as a predictor of worse quality of life measures and increased length of stay following spinal fusion. *World Neurosurg.* **2017**, *104*, 594–600. [CrossRef]
16. Neblett, R.; Cohen, H.; Choi, Y.; Hartzell, M.M.; Williams, M.; Mayer, T.G.; Gatchel, R.J. The central sensitization inventory (CSI): Establishing clinically significant values for identifiying central sensitivity syndromes in an outpatient chronic pain sample. *J. Pain* **2013**, *14*, 438–445. [CrossRef]
17. dos Santos Proença, J.; Baad-Hansen, L.; do Vale Braido, G.V.; Mercante, F.G.; Campi, L.B.; de Godoi Gonçalves, D.A. Lack of correlation between central sensitization and psychophysical measures of central sensitization in individuals with painful temporomandibular disorder. *Arch. Oral Biol. Biol.* **2021**, *124*, 105063. [CrossRef]
18. Hendriks, E.; Voogt, L.; Lenoir, D.; Coppieters, I.; Ickmans, K. Convergent validity of the central sensitization inventory in chronic whiplash-associated disorders; associations with quantitative sensory testing, pain intensity, fatigue, and psychosocial factors. *Pain Med.* **2020**, *21*, 3401–3412. [CrossRef]
19. Kregel, J.; Schumacher, C.; Dolphens, M.; Malfliet, A.; Goubert, D.; Lenoir, D.; Cagnie, B.; Meeus, M.; Coppieters, I. Convergent Validity of the dutch Central Sensitization Inventory: Associations with Psychophysical Pain Measures, Quality of life, Disability and Paun Cognitions in Patientes with Chronic spainal pain. *Pain Pract.* **2018**, *18*, 777–787. [CrossRef]
20. Rogelio, A.; Coronado, S.Z.G. The Central Sensitization Inventory and Pain Sensitivity Questionnaire: An Exploration of Construct Validity and Associations with Widespread Pain Sensitivity among Individuals with Shoulder Pain. *Musculoskelet. Care* **2018**, *36*, 61–67. [CrossRef]
21. Gervais-Hupé, J.; Pollice, J.; Sadi, J.; Carlesso, L.C. Validity of the central sensitization inventory with measures of sensitization in people with knee osteoarthritis. *Clin. Rheumatol.* **2018**, *37*, 3125–3132. [CrossRef]
22. Caumo, W.; Antunes, L.C.; Elkfury, J.L.; Herbstrith, E.G.; Sipmann, R.B.; Souza, A.; Torres, I.L.S.; Dos Santos, V.S.; Neblett, R. The central sensitization inventory validated and adapted for a Brazilian population: Psychometric properties and its relationship with brain-derived neurotrophic factor. *J. Pain Res.* **2017**, *10*, 2109–2122. [CrossRef]
23. Mikkonen, J.; Luomajoki, H.; Airaksinen, O.; Neblett, R.; Selander, T.; Leinonen, V. Cross-cultural adaptation and validation of the Finnish version of the central sensitization inventory and its relationship with dizziness and postural control. *BMC Neurol.* **2021**, *21*, 141. [CrossRef] [PubMed]
24. Basiri, K.; Katirji, B. Practical approach to electrodiagnosis of the carpal tunnel syndrome: A review. *Adv. Biomed. Res.* **2015**, *4*, 50. [CrossRef]
25. Levine, D.W.; Simmons, B.P.; Koris, M.J.; Daltroy, L.H.; Hohl, G.G.; Fossel, A.H.; Katz, J.N. A self-administered questionnaire for the assessment of severity of symptoms and functional status in carpal tunnel syndrome. *J. Bone Jt. Surg. Am.* **1993**, *75*, 1585–1592. [CrossRef]
26. Oteo-Álvaro, Á.; Marín, M.T.; Matas, J.A.; Vaquero, J. Validación al castellano de la escala Boston Carpal Tunnel Questionnaire. *Med. Clin.* **2016**, *146*, 247–253. [CrossRef]
27. Perez, C.; Galvez, R.; Huelbes, S.; Insausti, J.; Bouhassira, D.; Diaz, S.; Rejas, J. Validity and reliability of the Spanish version of the DN4 (Douleur Neuropathique 4 questions) questionnaire for differential diagnosis of pain syndromes associated to a neuropathic or somatic component. *Health Qual. Life Outcomes* **2007**, *5*, 66. [CrossRef]

28. Bouhassira, D.; Attal, N.; Alchaar, H.; Boureau, F.; Brochet, B.; Bruxelle, J.; Cunin, G.; Fermanian, J.; Ginies, P.; Grun-Overdyking, A.; et al. Comparison of pain syndromes associated with nervous or somatic lesions and development of a new neuropathic pain diagnostic questionnaire (DN4). *Pain* **2005**, *114*, 29–36. [CrossRef]
29. Cuesta-Vargas, A.I.; Roldan-Jimenez, C.; Neblett, R.; Gatchel, R.J. Cross-cultural adaptation and validity of the Spanish central sensitization inventory. *Springerplus* **2016**, *5*, 1837. [CrossRef]
30. Lacourt, T.E.; Houtveen, J.H.; van Doornen, L.J.P. Experimental pressure-pain assessments: Test-retest reliability, convergence and dimensionality. *Scand. J. Pain* **2012**, *3*, 31–37. [CrossRef]
31. Foucher, K.C.; Chmell, S.J.; Courtney, C.A. Duration of symptoms is associated with conditioned pain modulation and somatosensory measures in knee osteoarthritis. *J. Orthop. Res.* **2019**, *37*, 136–142. [CrossRef] [PubMed]
32. Tuveson, B.; Leffler, A.-S.; Hansson, P. Time dependant differences in pain sensitivity during unilateral ischemic pain provocation in healthy volunteers. *Eur. J. Pain* **2006**, *10*, 225. [CrossRef]
33. Nie, H.; Arendt-nielsen, L.; Andersen, H.; Graven-nielsen, T. Temporal Summation of Pain Evoked by Mechanical Stimulation in Deep and Superficial Tissue. *J. Pain* **2005**, *6*, 348–355. [CrossRef] [PubMed]
34. Katz, J.N.; Stirrat, C.R.; Larson, M.G.; Fossel, A.H.; Eaton, H.M.; Liang, M.H. A self-administered hand symptom diagram for the diagnosis and epidemiologic study of carpal tunnel syndrome. *J. Rheumatol.* **1990**, *17*, 1495–1498.
35. Beck, I.; Steer, R.A. Psychometric Properties of the Beck Depression Inventory: Twenty-Five Years of Evaluation. *Clin. Psychol. Rev.* **1988**, *8*, 77–100. [CrossRef]
36. Vega-Dienstmaier, J.; Coronado-Molina, Ó.; Mazzotti, G. Validez de una versión en español del Inventario de Depresión de Beck en pacientes hospitalizados de medicina general. *Rev. Neuropsiquiatr.* **2014**, *77*, 95. [CrossRef]
37. Guillén-Riquelme, A.; Buela-Casal, G. Psychometric revision and differential item functioning in the State Trait Anxiety Inventory (STAI). *Psicothema* **2011**, *23*, 510–515.
38. Gómez-Pérez, L.; López-Martínez, A.E.; Ruiz-Párraga, G.T. Psychometric Properties of the Spanish Version of the Tampa Scale for Kinesiophobia (TSK). *J. Pain* **2011**, *12*, 425–435. [CrossRef]
39. Hapidou, E.G.; O'Brien, M.A.; Pierrynowski, M.R.; de Las Heras, E.; Patel, M.; Patla, T. Fear and Avoidance of Movement in People with Chronic Pain: Psychometric Properties of the 11-Item Tampa Scale for Kinesiophobia (TSK-11). *Physiother. Can.* **2012**, *64*, 235–241. [CrossRef]
40. Faul, F.; Erdfelder., E.; Lang, A.-G.; Buchner, A. G*Power 3: A flexible statistical power analysis program for the social, behavioral, and biomedical sciences. *J. Mater. Environ. Sci.* **2007**, *39*, 175–191. [CrossRef]
41. de la Llave-Rincón, A.I.; Fernández-de-las-Peñas, C.; Laguarta-Val, S.; Alonso-Blanco, C.; Martínez-Perez, A.; Arendt-Nielsen, L.; Pareja, J.A. Increased Pain Sensitivity Is Not Associated with Electrodiagnostic Findings in Women with Carpal Tunnel Syndrome. *Clin. J. Pain* **2011**, *27*, 747–754. [CrossRef] [PubMed]
42. Matesanz, L.; Hausheer, A.C.; Baskozos, G.; Bennett, D.L.H.; Schmid, A.B. Somatosensory and psychological phenotypes associated with neuropathic pain in entrapment neuropathy. *Pain* **2021**, *162*, 1211–1220. [CrossRef] [PubMed]
43. Zanette, G.; Cacciatori, C.; Tamburin, S. Central sensitization in carpal tunnel syndrome with extraterritorial spread of sensory symptoms. *Pain* **2010**, *148*, 227–236. [CrossRef] [PubMed]
44. Baron, R.; Maier, C.; Attal, N.; Binder, A.; Bouhassira, D.; Cruccu, G.; Kennedy, J.D.; Magerl, W.; Mainka, T.; Reimer, M.; et al. Peripheral neuropathic pain: A mechanism-related organizing principle based on sensory profiles. *Pain* **2017**, *158*, 261–272. [CrossRef]
45. Baumann, K.; Simone, A.; Shain, N.; Lamotte, H. Neurogenic Hyperalgesia: The Search for the Primary Cutaneous Merent Fibers That Contribute to Capsaicin-Induced Pain and Hyperalgesia. *J. Neurophysiol.* **1991**, *66*, 212–227. [CrossRef]
46. Held, M.; Karl, F.; Vlckova, E.; Rajdova, A.; Escolano-Lozano, F.; Stetter, C.; Bharti, R.; Förstner, K.U.; Leinders, M.; Dušek, L.; et al. Sensory profiles and immune-related expression patterns of patients with and without neuropathic pain after peripheral nerve lesion. *Pain* **2019**, *160*, 2316–2327. [CrossRef]
47. Baskozos, G.; Sandy-hindmarch, O.; Clark, A.J.; Windsor, K.; Karlsson, P.; Weir, G.A.; Mcdermott, L.A.; Burchall, J.; Wiberg, A.; Furniss, D.; et al. Molecular and cellular correlates of human nerve regeneration: ADCYAP1/PACAP enhance nerve outgrowth. *Brain* **2020**, *143*, 2009–2026. [CrossRef]
48. Schmid, A.B.; Bland, J.D.P.; Bhat, M.A.; Bennett, D.L.H. The relationship of nerve fibre pathology to sensory function in entrapment neuropathy. *Brain* **2014**, *137*, 3186–3199. [CrossRef]
49. Raputova, J.; Srotova, I.; Vlckova, E.; Sommer, C.; Üçeyler, N.; Birklein, F.; Rittner, H.L.; Rebhorn, C.; Adamova, B.; Kovalova, I.; et al. Sensory phenotype and risk factors for painful diabetic neuropathy: A cross-sectional observational study. *Pain* **2017**, *158*, 2340–2353. [CrossRef]
50. Themistocleous, A.C.; Ramirez, J.D.; Shillo, P.R.; Lees, J.G.; Selvarajah, D.; Orengo, C.; Tesfaye, S.; Rice, A.S.C.; Bennett, D.L.H. The Pain in Neuropathy Study (PiNS): A cross-sectional observational study determining the somatosensory phenotype of painful and painless diabetic neuropathy. *Pain* **2016**, *157*, 1132–1145. [CrossRef]
51. Tampin, B.; Vollert, J.; Schmid, A.B. Sensory profiles are comparable in patients with distal and proximal entrapment neuropathies, while the pain experience differs. *Curr. Med. Res. Opin.* **2018**, *34*, 1899–1906. [CrossRef]
52. Neblett, R.; Hartzell, M.M.; Cohen, H.; Mayer, T.G.; Williams, M.; Choi, Y.H.; Gatchel, R.J. Ability of the central sensitization inventory to identify central sensitivity syndromes in an outpatient chronic pain sample. *Clin. J. Pain* **2015**, *31*, 323–332. [CrossRef]

53. Zafereo, J.; Wang-Price, S.; Kandil, E. Quantitative Sensory Testing Discriminates Central Sensitization Inventory Scores in Participants with Chronic Musculoskeletal Pain: An Exploratory Study. *Pain Pract.* **2021**, *21*, 547–556. [CrossRef]
54. Scerbo, T.; Colasurdo, J.; Dunn, S.; Unger, J.; Nijs, J.; Cook, C. Measurement Properties of the Central Sensitization Inventory: A Systematic Review. *Pain Pract.* **2018**, *18*, 544–554. [CrossRef]
55. Arendt-Nielsen, L.; Morlion, B.; Perrot, S.; Dahan, A.; Dickenson, A.; Kress, H.G.; Wells, C.; Bouhassira, D.; Mohr Drewes, A. Assessment and manifestation of central sensitisation across different chronic pain conditions. *Eur. J. Pain* **2018**, *22*, 216–241. [CrossRef]
56. Attal, N.; Lanteri-Minet, M.; Laurent, B.; Fermanian, J.; Bouhassira, D. The specific disease burden of neuropathic pain: Results of a French nationwide survey. *Pain* **2011**, *152*, 2836–2843. [CrossRef]
57. Oteo-Álvaro, Á.; Marín, M.T. Predictive factors of the neuropathic pain in patients with carpal tunnel syndrome and its impact on patient activity. *Pain Manag.* **2018**, *8*, 455–463. [CrossRef]
58. Portela, D.A.; Otero, P.E.; Biondi, M.; Romano, M.; Citi, S.; Mannucci, T.; Briganti, A.; Breghi, G.; Bollini, C. Peripheral nerve stimulation under ultrasonographic control to determine the needle-to-nerve relationship. *Vet. Anaesth. Analg.* **2013**, *40*, e91–e99. [CrossRef]
59. Van Griensven, H.; Schimd, A.; Trendafilova, T.; Low, M. Central sensitization in musculoskeletal pain: Lost in translation? *J. Orthop. Sports Phys. Ther.* **2020**, *50*, 592–596. [CrossRef]
60. Shetty, K.D.; Robbins, M.; Aragaki, D.; Basu, A.; Conlon, C.; Dworsky, M.; Benner, D.; Seelam, R.; Nuckols, T.K. The quality of electrodiagnostic tests for carpal tunnel syndrome: Implications for surgery, outcomes, and expenditures. *Muscle Nerve* **2020**, *62*, 60–69. [CrossRef]
61. Enax-Krumova, E.; Attal, N.; Bouhassira, D.; Freynhagen, R.; Gierthmühlen, J.; Hansson, P.; Kuehler, B.; Maier, C.; Sachau, J.; Segerdahl, M.; et al. Contralateral Sensory and Pain Perception Changes in Patients with Unilateral Neuropathy. *Neurology* **2021**, *97*, e389–e402. [CrossRef]
62. Petersen, K.K.; Vaegter, H.B.; Stubhaug, A.; Wolff, A.; Scammell, B.E.; Arendt-Nielsen, L.; Larsen, D.B. The predictive value of quantitative sensory testing: A systematic review on chronic postoperative pain and the analgesic effect of pharmacological therapies in patients with chronic pain. *Pain* **2021**, *162*, 31–44. [CrossRef]
63. Baron, R.; Förster, M.; Binder, A. Subgrouping of patients with neuropathic pain according to pain-related sensory abnormalities: A first step to a stratified treatment approach. *Lancet Neurol.* **2012**, *11*, 999–1005. [CrossRef]
64. Yarnitsky, D.; Granot, M.; Nahman-Averbuch, H.; Khamaisi, M.; Granovsky, Y. Conditioned pain modulation predicts duloxetine efficacy in painful diabetic neuropathy. *Pain* **2012**, *153*, 1193–1198. [CrossRef]
65. Petersen, K.K.; Simonsen, O.; Olesen, A.E.; Mørch, C.D.; Arendt-Nielsen, L. Pain inhibitory mechanisms and response to weak analgesics in patients with knee osteoarthritis. *Eur. J. Pain* **2019**, *23*, 1904–1912. [CrossRef]
66. Bosma, R.L.; Cheng, J.C.; Rogachov, A.; Kim, J.A.; Hemington, K.S.; Osborne, N.R.; Raghavan, L.V.; Bhatia, A.; Davis, K.D. Brain dynamics and temporal summation of pain predicts neuropathic pain relief from ketamine infusion. *Anesthesiology* **2018**, *129*, 1015–1024. [CrossRef]
67. O'Leary, H.; Smart, K.M.; Moloney, N.A.; Doody, C.M. Nervous System Sensitization as a Predictor of Outcome in the Treatment of Peripheral Musculoskeletal Conditions: A Systematic Review. *Pain Pract.* **2017**, *17*, 249–266. [CrossRef]
68. van Helvoort, E.M.; Welsing, P.M.J.; Jansen, M.P.; Gielis, W.P.; Loef, M.; Kloppenburg, M.; Blanco, F.; Haugen, I.K.; Berenbaum, F.; Bay-Jensen, A.-C.; et al. Neuropathic pain in the IMI-APPROACH knee osteoarthritis cohort: Prevalence and phenotyping. *RMD Open* **2021**, *7*, e002025. [CrossRef]

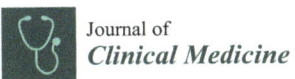 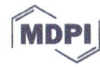

Article

The Accuracy of a Screening System for Carpal Tunnel Syndrome Using Hand Drawing

Takuro Watanabe [1,†], Takafumi Koyama [2,†], Eriku Yamada [2], Akimoto Nimura [3], Koji Fujita [3,*] and Yuta Sugiura [1]

1 School of Science for Open and Environmental Systems, Graduate School of Science and Technology, Keio University, Kanagawa 223-8522, Japan; t-tawatana@keio.jp (T.W.); sugiura@keio.jp (Y.S.)
2 Department of Orthopedic and Spinal Surgery, Graduate School of Medical and Dental Sciences, Tokyo Medical and Dental University, Tokyo 113-8510, Japan; koya.orth@tmd.ac.jp (T.K.); erikorth@tmd.ac.jp (E.Y.)
3 Department of Functional Joint Anatomy, Graduate School of Medical and Dental Sciences, Tokyo Medical and Dental University, Tokyo 113-8510, Japan; nimura.orj@tmd.ac.jp
* Correspondence: fujiorth@tmd.ac.jp; Tel.: +81-3-5803-5279
† Both authors contributed equally.

Abstract: When carpal tunnel syndrome (CTS), an entrapment neuropathy, becomes severe, thumb motion is reduced, which affects manual dexterity, such as causing difficulties in writing; therefore, early detection of CTS by screening is desirable. To develop a screening method for CTS, we developed a tablet app to measure the stylus trajectory and pressure of the stylus tip when drawing a spiral on a tablet screen using a stylus and, subsequently, used these data as training data to predict the classification of participants as non-CTS or CTS patients using a support vector machine. We recruited 33 patients with CTS and 31 healthy volunteers for this study. From our results, non-CTS and CTS were classified by our screening method with 82% sensitivity and 71% specificity. Our CTS screening method can facilitate the screening for potential patients with CTS and provide a quantitative assessment of CTS.

Keywords: carpal tunnel syndrome; support vector machine; machine learning; tablet app; screening; manual dexterity; drawing; nerve; pain; mobility

Citation: Watanabe, T.; Koyama, T.; Yamada, E.; Nimura, A.; Fujita, K.; Sugiura, Y. The Accuracy of a Screening System for Carpal Tunnel Syndrome Using Hand Drawing. J. Clin. Med. 2021, 10, 4437. https://doi.org/10.3390/jcm10194437

Academic Editor: Christian Carulli

Received: 4 September 2021
Accepted: 24 September 2021
Published: 27 September 2021

Publisher's Note: MDPI stays neutral with regard to jurisdictional claims in published maps and institutional affiliations.

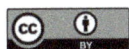

Copyright: © 2021 by the authors. Licensee MDPI, Basel, Switzerland. This article is an open access article distributed under the terms and conditions of the Creative Commons Attribution (CC BY) license (https://creativecommons.org/licenses/by/4.0/).

1. Introduction

Carpal tunnel syndrome (CTS) is one of the most common entrapment neuropathies [1]. The initial symptoms are numbness and sensory disturbance from the thumb to the ring finger; however, because these subjective symptoms do not significantly disrupt their daily activities, the patients do not seek medical attention [2]. As the severity of CTS increases, there is a possible failure of thumb motion, and the patients undergo carpal tunnel release surgery [3], which increases their physical burden. Furthermore, the postoperative outcome is poor and in some severe cases [4]. Conservative treatments of CTS, such as oral medications, injections, and wrist support, are expected to be effective if initiated at the early stage of CTS; therefore, early detection of CTS by screening is desirable.

Accordingly, mobile apps [5,6] have been developed to serve as a simple and objective screening tool for CTS. These apps have focused on the failure of thumb motion caused by atrophy of the thenar muscle, which affects manual dexterity, causing patients to be aware of associated symptoms, such as difficulties in fastening their buttons and writing [7]. In particular, writing plays an important role in our daily lives; therefore, it is significantly impacted by the failure of the thumb motion.

Recent advances in sensing technology have proposed pens and motion capture tools that can measure writing motion [8,9]. However, previous studies could not set up an experimental environment to measure writing motion because of the special devices and systems required. Thus, there have been attempts to evaluate writing motion using off-the-shelf tablets and styluses [10]. Since tablets can measure handwriting pressure and altitude–azimuth of styluses, tablet apps have been developed to evaluate writing motion in dysgraphia [11] and Parkinson's disease [12]. Moreover, the use of off-the-shelf devices not only reduces the cost of preparing special experimental environments, but also reduces medical costs as a result of the early detection of diseases outside of medical institutions, such as at home [13–16].

We hypothesized that sensory disturbance and the lack of manual dexterity, resulting from CTS, affect stylus manipulation, and we developed a screening method for CTS, focusing on drawing motion, using a tablet and stylus and verified for its accuracy (Figure 1a).

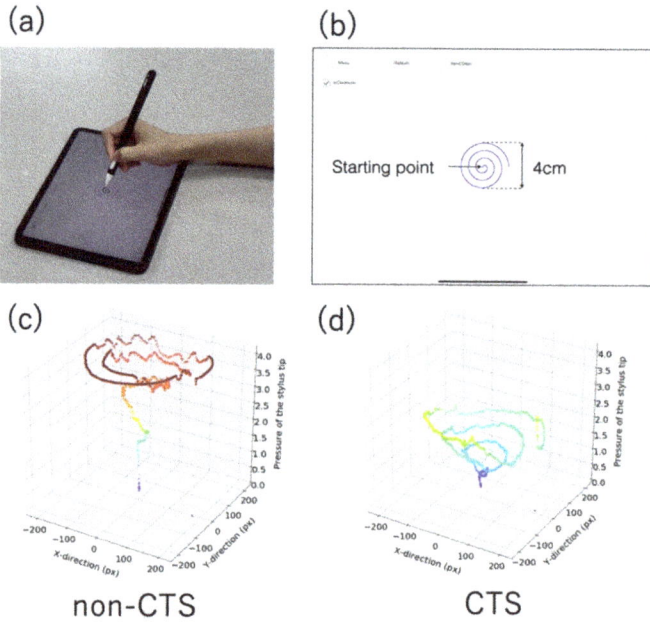

Figure 1. (a) A participant using the stylus on the app installed on the tablet. (b) The app screen. Participants drew a spiral along the blue guide spiral. The longitudinal diameter of the guide spiral was set to 4 cm to observe their manual dexterity. (c,d) are 3D graphs with the stylus trajectory on the xy-plane and the pressure of the stylus tip on the vertical axis drawn by non-CTS and CTS participants, respectively.

2. Materials and Methods

This study was approved by the Institutional Review Board of Tokyo Medical and Dental University. Informed consent was obtained from all the participants.

2.1. Participants

We recruited 33 patients with CTS and 31 healthy volunteers from July 2020 to March 2021. The CTS group was diagnosed with CTS by hand surgeons in the orthopedic outpatient clinic based on physical examinations and nerve conduction studies. The nerve conduction study, including motor and sensory nerve conduction velocity studies, was performed using Neuropack X1 (Nihon Kohden, Tokyo, Japan). The results were used to classify the severity of CTS based on the Bland classification [17]. The patients with CTS answered the Disabilities of the Arm, Shoulder, and Hand (DASH) questionnaire [18]. The score for question 2 on writing was extracted from the DASH score and recorded as the DASH score (writing) on a scale of 1–5, with 5 indicating the highest degree of writing disability. In addition, their pulp pinch strength and grip strength were measured. The non-CTS group comprised patients who had visited the orthopedic outpatient clinic or had been hospitalized for conditions other than CTS and had no hand complaints or abnormal findings upon examination by the hand surgeons. Participants with a history of upper extremity disease, injury, or surgery; those with inflammatory diseases such as rheumatoid arthritis; those with neurological diseases such as stroke, cervical myelopathy, and radiculopathy; and those with psychiatric diseases were excluded from both groups because these diseases affect hand movement. All the participants were right hand dominant; therefore, they manipulated the stylus with their right hand. The participants sat on a 40 cm high chair and placed the tablet on a 70 cm high desk. While drawing, the elbows and ulnar sides of the hands rested on the desk and the tablet. They drew three spirals, and the last of the three was analyzed.

2.2. App Design

We developed a tablet app to measure the trajectory and pressure of the stylus tip when drawing a spiral on a tablet screen using a stylus (Figure 1a). A blue guide spiral was drawn on the app screen, and the participants used the stylus to draw another spiral along the guide spiral (Figure 1b). As examples, 3D graphs with the stylus trajectory on the xy-plane and the pressure of the stylus tip on the vertical axis for non-CTS and CTS participants are shown in Figure 1c,d, respectively. The longitudinal diameter of the guide spiral was set to 4 cm to observe their manual dexterity and is expressed by the polar equation,

$$r = -\theta \ (0 \leq \theta \leq 7\pi) \tag{1}$$

where r and θ represent radius and angle, respectively. After measuring the trajectory and pressure of the stylus tip, the data were transferred to Elasticsearch (version 7.4, Elastic, Amsterdam, The Netherlands) deployed on Amazon Web Service.

We used a 1st generation iPad Pro 11" (Apple, Cupertino, CA, USA) and 2nd generation Apple Pencil (Apple, Cupertino, USA), which were among the most popular tablets and styluses available at the time. The frame rate of the tablet screen was 120 fps, and the range of the pressure of the stylus tip was between 0 and 4.166667, which was the custom unit defined by the tablet's operating system. To improve the drawing comfort and grip of the Apple Pencil, we attached a Pencil Barrier 2 (JJT, Tokyo, Japan) to the Apple Pencil and a paper-like film (MS factory, Kyoto, Japan) to the screen. The app was developed using Unity (version 2019.2.17f1, Unity Technologies, San Francisco, USA).

2.3. CTS Classification Using a Support Vector Machine

We created a two-class classification model, non-CTS and CTS, using a support vector machine (SVM) [19], based on the data obtained from the app we developed. To classify patients into the non-CTS or CTS groups, we prepared four training data points for the SVM (Table 1).

Table 1. Prepared training data for the support vector machine.

Index	Training Data	Dimension
①	Jerk of the pressure of the stylus tip	256
②	Jerk of the trajectory of the stylus tip	256
③	RMSE [1] between the participant's spiral and the model spiral	1
④	Maximum pressure of the stylus tip	1

[1] RMSE: root mean square error

2.4. The Jerk of the Trajectory and Pressure of the Stylus Tip

We preprocessed time-series data of the trajectory and pressure of the stylus tip measured by the app we developed (Figure 2) and used them as training data for the SVM.

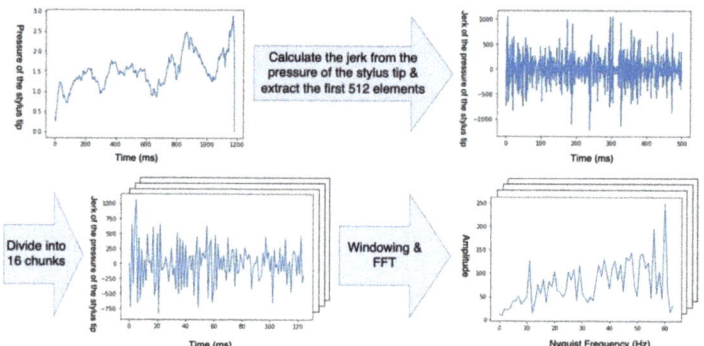

Figure 2. We calculated the jerk from the time-series data of pressure of the stylus tip and extracted the first 512 elements, then applied the Hanning window function and fast Fourier transform (FFT). Finally, the Nyquist frequency, which is half of the sampling frequency, was used as training data.

Firstly, we calculated the jerk from the trajectory and that from the pressure of the stylus tip for each participant. This was because the velocity of the stylus movement and the pressure of the stylus tip differed among the participants. The sampling frequency was 120 Hz. The first 512 frames were extracted from each jerk due to the following two reasons: The first was to enable a classification independent of the time used to draw the spiral—all the participants used more than 5 s to complete the drawing; therefore, we obtained data on a duration less than 5 s for any participants (Figure 3). The second reason was to ensure a quick computation of the fast Fourier transform (FFT) described below when the number of data points is a power of two [20]. We divided the 512 frames into 16 chunks; thus, each chunk consisted of data from 32 frames. Finally, we obtained the frequency components by applying the Hanning window function and FFT to each chunk. Each chunk was converted into 32 frequency components. According to the Nyquist–Shannon sampling theorem, frequency components of up to 60 Hz, which was half of the sampling frequency, were used as the training data. At the end of the training, a 256-dimension dataset (16 chunks × 16 frequency components) was obtained for each participant.

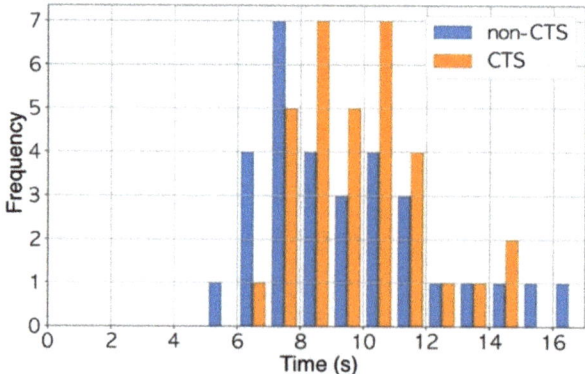

Figure 3. All participants took at least 5 s to complete the drawing.

2.5. Root Mean Square Error between the Participants' Spirasl and the Model Spiral

We calculated the root mean square error (RMSE) between the spirals drawn by the participants and the model spiral. The spiral was not in the Cartesian coordinate system (Figure 4a) but was transformed into a polar coordinate system with θ ($0 \leq \theta \leq 2\pi$) to simplify the observation. We then obtained the spiral plotted with θ on the horizontal axis and r on the vertical axis (Figure 4b) and calculated the RMSE.

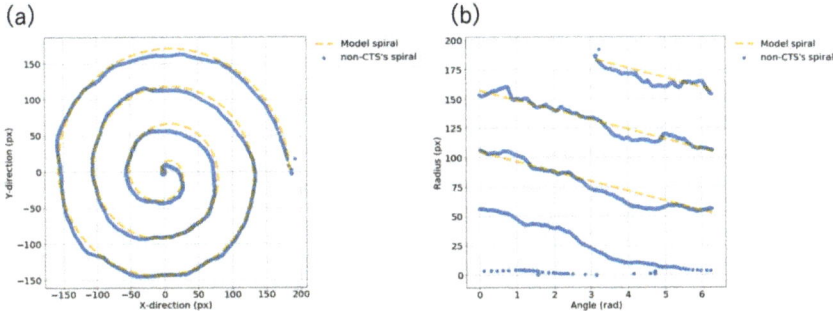

Figure 4. (a) Spiral plotted in the Cartesian coordinate system. (b) Spiral plotted with θ on the horizontal axis and r on the vertical axis. The solid line is the spiral drawn by a non-CTS participant, and the dashed line is the model spiral. We calculated the root mean square error between the solid and dashed lines.

The section from the start of the spiral to 2π was excluded from the observation area. This was because when the participants started drawing from a position off the starting point, noise was generated (Figure 4b). We tried to eliminate this noise by using thresholds of θ and r, but this was difficult because the noise generated was different for each participant.

2.6. Statistical Analysis

We used a two-tailed Student's t-test to compare the age in years of the participants and a Chi-square test to compare sex between the non-CTS and CTS groups. The CTS group was divided into patients with grades 1–3 and those with grades 4–6 based on the Bland classification [17], and we compared DASH score, DASH score (writing), pulp pinch strength, grip strength, and disease duration between the patients with grades 1–3 and those with grades 4–6 using the Mann–Whitney U test. The RMSE between the spiral drawn by the participants and the model spiral and the maximum pressure of the stylus tip between the non-CTS and CTS groups were compared using the Mann–Whitney U test. In addition, we compared their data between the patients with grades 1–3 and those with grades 4–6. A p value of ≤ 0.05 was considered a statistically significant difference.

Regarding the SVM, leave-one-out cross-validation was used for classification accuracy verification. The hyperparameters, such as the degree of the kernel function and regularization parameter, for the SVM were tuned so that the cutoff values of the receiver operating characteristic curves were close to the upper left of the graphs.

Our analyses were performed using Python (version 3.7.3, Python Software Foundation) and a machine learning library, scikit-learn (version 0.21.3, scikit-learn developers).

3. Results

3.1. Participant Characteristics

The characteristics of the participants are summarized in Tables 2 and 3. There was no significant difference in age and sex between the non-CTS and CTS groups. Between the patients with grades 1–3 and those with grades 4–6, only DASH score (writing) was significantly higher in the patients with grades 4–6; there was no significant difference in the other characteristics.

Table 2. Characteristics of participants in the CTS and non-CTS groups.

Participant Characteristics	Non-CTS [1] Group	CTS Group	p Value
Number of participants, N	31	33	N/A [2]
Sex (female), n (%)	18 (58.1)	26 (78.8)	0.074
Age in years, median (IQR [3])	64 (55–72)	67 (60–73)	0.280
Bland classification			
Grade 1	N/A	1	
Grade 2	N/A	4	
Grade 3	N/A	15	
Grade 4	N/A	1	
Grade 5	N/A	10	
Grade 6	N/A	2	

[1] CTS: carpal tunnel syndrome. [2] N/A: not applicable. [3] IQR: interquartile range.

Table 3. Characteristics of participants in the CTS group, CTS grades 1–3, and grades 4–6.

Participant Characteristics	CTS [1] Group	Grades 1–3	Grades 4–6	p Value
DASH score, mean (SD [2])	26.6 (19.4)	24.4 (22.2)	29.7 (13.9)	0.300
DASH score (writing), mean (SD)	1.8 (1.0)	1.4 (0.8)	2.3 (1.0)	0.005
Pulp pinch strength (kg), mean (SD)	2.6 (1.5)	3.0 (1.6)	2.1 (1.0)	0.082
Grip strength (kg), mean (SD)	17.3 (8.8)	18.1 (9.7)	16.2 (7.2)	0.807
Disease duration (year), mean (SD)	2.6 (2.6)	2.7 (2.6)	2.4 (2.6)	0.797

[1] CTS: carpal tunnel syndrome. [2] SD: standard deviation

3.2. Root Mean Square Error between the Participants' Spirals and the Model Spiral

There were significant differences in the RMSE between the participant's spiral and the model spiral between the non-CTS and CTS groups (Figure 5a) and between patients with CTS grades 1–3 and those with grades 4–6 (Figure 6a).

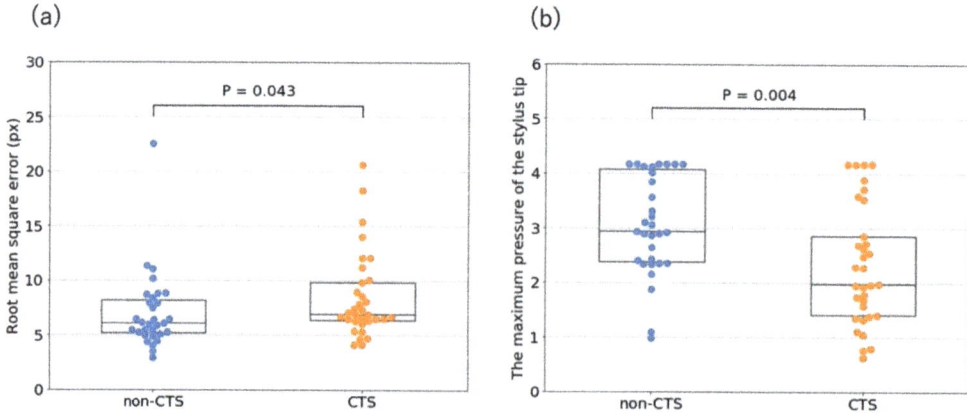

Figure 5. (**a**) Comparison of root mean square errors between the participants' spirals and the model spiral in the non-CTS and CTS groups. (**b**) Comparison of the maximum pressures of the stylus tip between the non-CTS and CTS groups. There were significant differences between the non-CTS and CTS groups in each comparison.

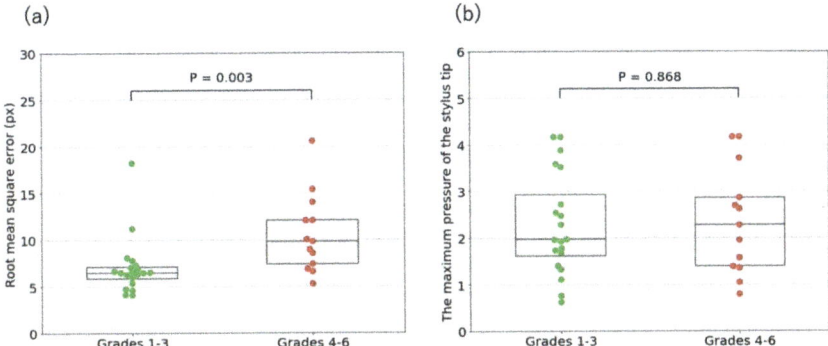

Figure 6. The CTS group was divided into two groups, patients with CTS grades 1–3 and those with CTS grades 4–6, based on the Bland classification. (**a**) Comparison of root mean square errors between the participants' spirals and the model spiral in the patients with CTS grades 1–3 and those with CTS grades 4–6. There was a significant difference between the grades. (**b**) Comparison of the maximum pressures of the stylus tip between patients with CTS grades 1–3 and those with CTS grades 4–6.

3.3. Maximum Pressure of the Stylus Tip

There were significant differences in the maximum pressure of the stylus tip between the non-CTS and CTS groups (Figure 5b). Contrarily, there was no significant difference in the maximum pressure between patients with CTS grades 1–3 and those with CTS grades 4–6 (Figure 6b).

3.4. CTS Classification Using a Support Vector Machine

The classification using the data from the jerk of the trajectory of the stylus tip as training data showed the highest sensitivity, while the classification using the data from the jerk of the pressure of the stylus tip as training data showed the highest specificity (Tables 1 and 4 and Figure 7).

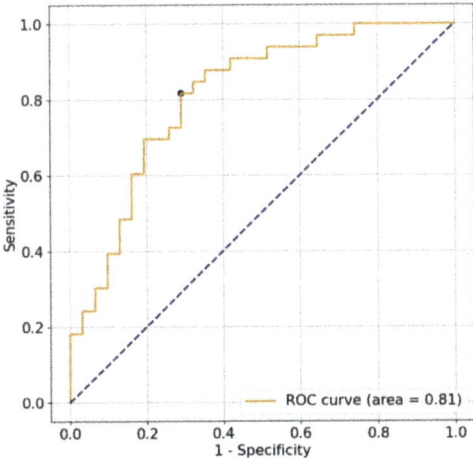

Figure 7. The receiver operating characteristic curve for classification using the jerk of the trajectory of the stylus tip. The sensitivity and specificity were 82% and 71%, respectively, when the cutoff was the black point closest to the upper left of the graph. The area under the curve was 0.81.

Table 4. Classification results of indices of training data described in Table 1.

Training Data	Sensitivity, %	Specificity, %	Accuracy, %	AUC [1]
①	76	77	77	0.77
②	82	71	77	0.81
③	61	65	63	0.58
④	73	65	69	0.58
① + ②	73	81	77	0.79
① + ③	76	77	77	0.77
① + ④	76	77	77	0.77
② + ③	82	71	77	0.81
② + ④	82	71	77	0.81
③ + ④	58	84	70	0.70
① + ② + ③	73	81	77	0.79
① + ② + ④	73	81	77	0.79
① + ③ + ④	76	77	77	0.78
② + ③ + ④	82	71	77	0.81
① + ② + ③ + ④	73	81	77	0.79

[1] AUC: area under curve

4. Discussion

In this study, we developed a tablet app that measured the stylus trajectory and pressure of the stylus tip for CTS screening. The sensitivity and specificity of the classification based on the jerk of the stylus tip trajectory were 82% and 71%, respectively (Figure 7). The tablet app in our study did not show high sensitivity compared to that of a previous tablet app [5], which showed 93% sensitivity and 73% specificity, and to that of a previous smartphone app [6], which showed a sensitivity of 94% and specificity of 67%. Contrarily, our specificity was as high as that of the other apps. Previous screening apps [5,6] focused on the failure of the thumb motion caused by atrophy of the thenar muscle. We thought that the apps made it difficult for the patients to perform compensatory movements for the failure of the thumb motion, which was otherwise capable of expressing the characteristics of the failure sufficiently. In our study, in contrast, the flexor tendons of the index and middle fingers compensated for atrophy of the thenar muscle; therefore, it may not have been as well characterized as that of the apps, which was the reason why our sensitivity was not as high as that of the apps. However, as an advantage, our method does not require patients to learn a special game and only involves drawing spirals on a tablet screen, making it easy even for older adults who are not familiar with games. We believe that developing screening methods that require a variety of hand motions can help identify potential patients in the early stages of CTS.

The two sets of training data, the jerk of the trajectory and jerk of the pressure of the stylus tip, showed higher sensitivity and specificity in this study. This implies that our screening can be used if any of the data, the jerk of the trajectory or jerk of the pressure of the stylus tip, are available. Considering that cheap tablets cannot measure the pressure of the stylus tip but can measure the stylus trajectory, our app will help in identifying various patients with CTS because it works on cheap tablets.

Regarding the RMSE between the participants' spirals and the model spiral, there were significant differences between the non-CTS and CTS groups (Figure 5a), and between the patients with CTS grades 1–3 and those with CTS grades 4–6 (Figure 6a). Compared to the non-CTS group and patients with CTS grades 1–3, patients with CTS grades 4–6 had severe sensory disturbance in the hand and atrophy of the thenar muscle, which seemed to affect manual dexterity, such as accurate drawing. Contrarily, patients with CTS grades 1–3 had mild sensory disturbance and pain in the hand, which seemed not to affect accurate drawing. Additionally, 20 of the patients in the CTS group, comprising the majority, were classified as having CTS grades 1–3, which may explain why the RMSE did not contribute to the CTS classification.

A previous study [9] examined manual dexterity by comparing the maximum pressure of the stylus tip between the non-CTS and CTS groups and reported a significant difference between the groups. Our study also showed similar results (Figure 5b), but the maximum pressure of the stylus tip was higher in the non-CTS group than in the CTS group, which contradicts the observations in the previous study. This could be attributed to the different writing motion used in their study; their study participants drew Arabic numerals, and in this study, the participants drew spirals. Since Arabic numerals are one of the characters that participants are accustomed to writing daily, there is a possibility that individual habits may interfere and may be falsely tagged as abnormal motion. Furthermore, the writing accuracy was not examined in the previous study, even though the participants traced the thinly written numerals with a pen, and it took time to evaluate the ten numerals. Therefore, referring to another previous study [21], we used spirals that would allow us to finish the test in a short time and generate consistent data. In addition, while the previous study [9] did not consider the severity of CTS, we attempted to explore the manual dexterity caused by CTS by classifying the severity. Finally, the previous study aimed to find indices of significant differences, while we aimed to develop a screening method, which is a critical difference between our study and efforts by others.

Additionally, there was no significant difference between the patients with CTS grades 1–3 and those with CTS grades 4–6 (Figure 6b), which meant severe sensory disturbance and atrophy of the thenar muscle did not affect the maximum pressure of the stylus tip. To maintain the pressure, the flexor tendons of the index and middle fingers may have compensated for atrophy of the thenar muscle [9]. Furthermore, forearm muscles may also have to do with the compensation.

Overall, our analyses implied that severe sensory disturbance and atrophy of the thenar muscle affected accurate drawing, but not pressure of the stylus tip.

This study has some limitations. It is difficult to use this screening method if users develop CTS in their non-dominant hands, since the non-dominant hand cannot draw as precisely as the dominant hand. Furthermore, this study only examined CTS and did not examine other diseases, such as cerebral infarction, cervical spondylosis, diabetic neuropathy, and cubital tunnel syndrome, which also cause a lack of manual dexterity. In addition, non-disease status, such as muscle weakness based on aging and non-painful joint deformity, may also affect manual dexterity; therefore, we will attempt to compare the findings before and after intervention (pre- and post-carpal tunnel release) to control for the confounding effects of these symptoms, making our method more reliable. This study examined this method of CTS screening by analyzing the spirals drawn by participants. In a future study, we will consider comparing the screening accuracy of other shapes, such as square and sine waves, and incorporate additional parameters, such as altitude–azimuth of styluses, into training data to improve the accuracy. Our aim is to provide a screening method for CTS with movements that fit our daily lives, such as writing one's name.

5. Conclusions

We developed a new tablet app, focusing on drawing motion, for CTS screening that measures the trajectory and pressure of the stylus tip when drawing a spiral with the stylus. Our method uses off-the-shelf tablets, which makes it easier to identify potential patients with CTS and enables quantitative assessment of CTS.

Author Contributions: Conceptualization, K.F.; methodology, software, formal analysis, and visualization, T.W.; data curation, T.K. and E.Y.; writing—original draft preparation, T.W.; writing—review and editing, K.F., T.K. and Y.S; supervision and project administration, K.F., Y.S. and A.N.; funding acquisition, Y.S. and K.F.; T.W. and T.K. contributed equally. All authors have read and agreed to the published version of the manuscript.

Funding: This research was funded by JST PRESTO, grant number JPMJPR17J4; JST AIP-PRISM, grant number JPMJCR18Y2; and JSPS KAKENHI, grant number JP21H03485.

Institutional Review Board Statement: This study was approved by the Institutional Review Board of Tokyo Medical and Dental University, approval number M2019-047, approved 25 June 2019.

Informed Consent Statement: Informed consent was obtained from all subjects involved in the study.

Data Availability Statement: The data generated in this study are available from the corresponding author on reasonable request.

Acknowledgments: We would like to thank Kaho Kato, Keio University, and Hayate Umemoto, Tokyo Medical and Dental University, for the data analyses.

Conflicts of Interest: The authors declare no conflict of interest.

References

1. Padua, L.; Coraci, D.; Erra, C.; Pazzaglia, C.; Paolasso, I.; Loreti, C.; Caliandro, P.; Hobson-Webb, L.D. Carpal tunnel syndrome: Clinical features, diagnosis, and management. *Lancet Neurol.* **2016**, *15*, 1273–1284. [CrossRef]
2. Fernandes, C.H.; Meirelles, L.M.; Raduan Neto, J.; Nakachima, L.R.; Dos Santos, J.B.; Faloppa, F. Carpal tunnel syndrome with thenar atrophy: Evaluation of the pinch and grip strength in patients undergoing surgical treatment. *Hand* **2013**, *8*, 60–63. [CrossRef] [PubMed]
3. De Kleermaeker, F.; Meulstee, J.; Bartels, R.; Verhagen, W. Long-term outcome after carpal tunnel release and identification of prognostic factors. *Acta Neurochir.* **2019**, *161*, 663–671. [CrossRef] [PubMed]
4. Rivlin, M.; Kachooei, A.R.; Wang, M.L.; Ilyas, A.M. Electrodiagnostic grade and carpal tunnel release outcomes: A prospective analysis. *J. Hand Surg. Am.* **2018**, *43*, 425–431. [CrossRef] [PubMed]
5. Fujita, K.; Watanabe, T.; Kuroiwa, T.; Sasaki, T.; Nimura, A.; Sugiura, Y. A tablet-based App for carpal tunnel syndrome screening: Diagnostic case-control study. *JMIR Mhealth Uhealth* **2019**, *7*, e14172. [CrossRef] [PubMed]
6. Koyama, T.; Sato, S.; Toriumi, T.; Watanabe, T.; Nimura, A.; Okawa, A.; Sugiura, Y.; Fujita, K. A screening method using anomaly detection on a smartphone for patients with carpal tunnel syndrome: Diagnostic case-control study. *JMIR Mhealth Uhealth* **2021**, *9*, e26320. [CrossRef] [PubMed]
7. Atroshi, I.; Gummesson, C.; Johnsson, R.; Sprinchorn, A. Symptoms, disability, and quality of life in patients with carpal tunnel syndrome. *J. Hand Surg. Am.* **1999**, *24*, 398–404. [CrossRef]
8. Fujisawa, Y.; Okajima, Y. Characteristics of handwriting of people with cerebellar ataxia: Three-dimensional movement analysis of the pen tip, finger, and wrist. *Phys. Ther.* **2015**, *95*, 1547–1558. [CrossRef] [PubMed]
9. Kuo, L.C.; Hsu, H.M.; Wu, P.T.; Lin, S.C.; Hsu, H.Y.; Jou, I.M. Impact of distal median neuropathy on handwriting performance for patients with carpal tunnel syndrome in office and administrative support occupations. *J. Occup. Rehabil.* **2014**, *24*, 332–343. [CrossRef] [PubMed]
10. Sisti, J.A.; Christophe, B.; Seville, A.R.; Garton, A.L.; Gupta, V.P.; Bandin, A.J.; Yu, Q.; Pullman, S.L. Computerized spiral analysis using the iPad. *J. Neurosci. Methods* **2017**, *275*, 50–54. [CrossRef] [PubMed]
11. Asselborn, T.; Chapatte, M.; Dillenbourg, P. Extending the spectrum of dysgraphia: A data driven strategy to estimate handwriting quality. *Sci. Rep.* **2020**, *10*, 1–11. [CrossRef] [PubMed]
12. Impedovo, D.; Pirlo, G. Dynamic handwriting analysis for the assessment of neurodegenerative diseases: A pattern recognition perspective. *IEEE Rev. Biomed. Eng.* **2018**, *12*, 209–220. [CrossRef] [PubMed]
13. Elgendi, M.; Fletcher, R.; Liang, Y.; Howard, N.; Lovell, N.H.; Abbott, D.; Lim, K.; Ward, R. The use of photoplethysmography for assessing hypertension. *NPJ Digit. Med.* **2019**, *2*, 1–11. [CrossRef] [PubMed]
14. Pamplona, V.; Ankit, M.; Oliveira, M.; Raskar, R. NETRA: Interactive display for estimating refractive errors and focal range. *ACM Trans. Graph.* **2010**, *29*, 1–8. [CrossRef]
15. Quinn, C.C.; Clough, S.S.; Minor, J.M.; Lender, D.; Okafor, M.C.; Gruber-Baldini, A. WellDoc mobile diabetes management randomized controlled trial: Change in clinical and behavioral outcomes and patient and physician satisfaction. *Diabetes Technol. Ther.* **2008**, *10*, 160–168. [CrossRef] [PubMed]
16. Liang, Y.; Fan, H.; Fang, Z.; Miao, L.; Li, W.; Zhang, Z.; Sun, W.; Wang, K.; He, L.; Chen, A. OralCam: Enabling self-examination and awareness of oral health using a smartphone camera. In Proceedings of the 2020 CHI Conference on Human Factors in Computing Systems, Honolulu, HI, USA, 25–30 April 2020.
17. Bland, J.D. A neurophysiological grading scale for carpal tunnel syndrome. *Muscle Nerve* **2000**, *23*, 1280–1283. [CrossRef]
18. Hudak, P.L.; Amadio, P.C.; Bombardier, C.; Beaton, D.; Cole, D.; Davis, A.; Hawker, G.; Katz, J.N.; Makela, M.; Marx, R.G.; et al. Development of an upper extremity outcome measure: The DASH (disabilities of the arm, shoulder, and hand). *Am. J. Ind. Med.* **1996**, *29*, 602–608. [CrossRef]
19. Boser, B.E.; Guyon, I.M.; Vapnik, V.N. A training algorithm for optimal margin classifiers. In Proceedings of the Fifth Annual Workshop on Computational Learning Theory, New York, NY, USA, 27–29 July 1992.

20. Cooley, J.W.; Tukey, J.W. An algorithm for the machine calculation of complex Fourier series. *Math. Comput.* **1965**, *19*, 297–301. [CrossRef]
21. San Luciano, M.; Wang, C.; Ortega, R.A.; Yu, Q.; Boschung, S.; Soto-Valencia, J.; Bressman, S.B.; Lipton, R.B.; Pullman, S.; Saunders-Pullman, R. Digitized spiral drawing: A possible biomarker for early parkinson's disease. *PLoS ONE* **2016**, *11*, e0162799. [CrossRef] [PubMed]

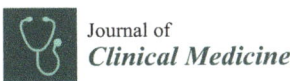

Review

Proximal Median Nerve Compression in the Differential Diagnosis of Carpal Tunnel Syndrome

Pekka Löppönen [1,*], Sina Hulkkonen [2] and Jorma Ryhänen [2]

1. Department of Orthopedics and Traumatology, Seinäjoki Central Hospital, FI-60220 Seinäjoki, Finland
2. Department of Hand Surgery, Helsinki University Hospital, University of Helsinki, FI-00029 Helsinki, Finland; sina.hulkkonen@hus.fi (S.H.); jorma.ryhanen@hus.fi (J.R.)
* Correspondence: pekka.lopponen@epshp.fi

Abstract: Carpal tunnel syndrome (CTS) is the most common median nerve compression neuropathy. Its symptoms and clinical presentation are well known. However, symptoms at median nerve distribution can also be caused by a proximal problem. Pronator syndrome (PS) and anterior interosseous nerve syndrome (AINS) with their typical characteristics have been thought to explain proximal median nerve problems. Still, the literature on proximal median nerve compressions (PMNCs) is conflicting, making this classic split too simple. This review clarifies that PMNCs should be understood as a spectrum of mild to severe nerve lesions along a branching median nerve, thus causing variable symptoms. Clear objective findings are not always present, and therefore, diagnosis should be based on a more thorough understanding of anatomy and clinical testing. Treatment should be planned according to each patient's individual situation. To emphasize the complexity of causes and symptoms, PMNC should be named proximal median nerve syndrome.

Keywords: carpal tunnel syndrome; median neuropathy; median nerve entrapment; neuralgic amyotrophy; pronator syndrome

1. Introduction

Carpal tunnel syndrome (CTS) is the most common median nerve compression neuropathy. As its clinical symptoms and presentation are well known, the correct diagnosis and treatment are evident. However, symptoms at median nerve distribution can also be caused by nerve compression proximal to the carpal tunnel. This should be remembered when symptoms are atypical to CTS or persist after carpal tunnel release (CTR).

Proximal median nerve compression (PMNC) is more uncommon than CTS and probably underdiagnosed. Diagnosis can be difficult due to overlapping symptoms with CTS; moreover, both can coexist in the same patient [1–6]. In addition, multiple anatomical features can cause entrapment of the median nerve, presenting various symptoms. Therefore, successful treatment of PMNC requires a thorough understanding of the median nerve's anatomical aspects, comprehension of its pathology and recovery, and experience interpreting the varying clinical presentations.

Only limited good-quality clinical research exists on PMNC. Most studies are small hospital-based series of surgically treated patients. No comparative trials have been published on treatment of PMNC. The largest problem with PMNC is the difficulty in differentiating whether or not it is a compressive neuropathy.

A literature search was performed in November 2021 in PubMed/Medline. Terms "Pronator syndrome", "Lacertus syndrome", "Supracondylar process syndrome", "Proximal median nerve compression", and "Anterior interosseous nerve syndrome" were used. Abstracts of published articles were read, and full-text versions were reviewed if they seemed relevant to the subject. All papers reporting data such as symptoms, clinical diagnosis, treatment, or outcome after treatment were selected. Articles focusing on only diagnostic studies and presenting no clinical features were not included. Only articles published in the English language were included. Only articles accessible at our facility were included.

The aim of this review is to summarize the existing literature on PMNC, examine the variations of this condition, identify related symptoms and signs, and help physicians in diagnosing and treating PMNC. This paper does not discuss median neuropathies more proximal in the shoulder such as cervical radiculopathy or thoracic outlet syndrome.

2. Anatomy and Sites of Median Nerve Compression

The literature is filled with different terminology representing a simplified understanding of the condition. The same diagnoses with different criteria have been accepted and used by many clinicians and authors. However, there are reasons why this traditional division should be reconsidered. Here, we guide the readers across the course of the median nerve and the compressive points and etiologies of PMNC discussed in the literature.

Median nerve fibers can be traced back to cervical roots of C5-C8 and thoracic root Th1. C5-C7 form the lateral cord, and C8 and Th1 form a smaller medial cord. Lateral and medial cords form the median nerve. The nerve then travels across the axilla and the medial side of the arm with the brachial artery between the biceps brachii and brachialis muscles.

2.1. Supracondylar Process, Ligament of Struthers, and Supracondylar Process Syndrome

Figure 1 shows the anatomy of the elbow. A supracondylar process or a bony spur about 3–6 cm proximal to the medial epicondyle is present in 1–2% of individuals. The ligament of Struthers is a fibrous arch between this process and the medial epicondyle [7], and the median nerve and brachial artery travel underneath it if it exists [8–10]. The median nerve can become compressed under this bony process or the ligament [9,11,12]. This neuropathy is known as supracondylar process syndrome [8,9,12,13]. The ligament of Struthers has been described to occur and cause compression of the median nerve even without the presence of a clinical supracondylar process [13–15].

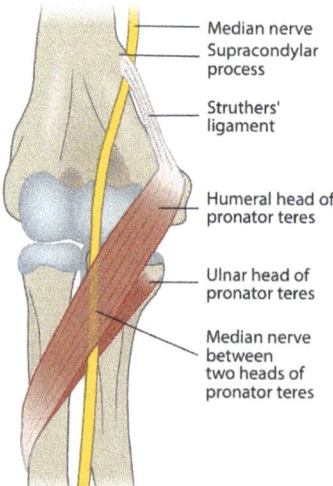

Figure 1. Course of the median nerve at the elbow.

2.2. Lacertus Fibrosus and Lacertus Syndrome

Bicipital aponeurosis or lacertus fibrosus originates from the biceps brachii muscle and joins the fascia of the pronator-flexor mass (Figure 2). The median nerve and brachial artery pass underneath and are prone to compression in forearm pronosupination [2,6,11,14–20]. Persisting median artery has also been described to cause median nerve compression [6].

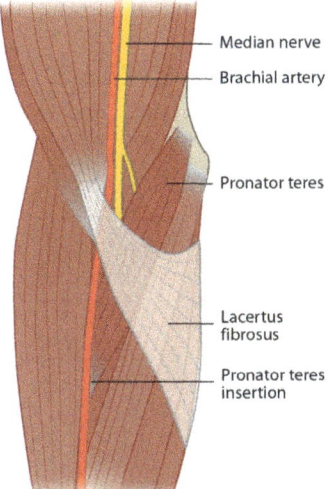

Figure 2. Lacertus fibrosus covers the pronator-flexor mass and the median nerve.

Lacertus syndrome (LS) and its symptoms in baseball pitchers were first described by Bennett in 1959 [21]. It has more recently been popularized by Hagert and Lalonde [22]. Symptoms of LS are described as a loss of key and pinch strength, loss of fine motor skills, and sense of clumsiness. Hagert states that patients with LS have (1) weakness in median nerve innervated muscles distal to lacertus fibrosus, (2) pain when compressing the nerve at the level of lacertus fibrosus, and (3) a positive scratch collapse test. These patients rarely have paresthesia in the median nerve innervated hand [23]. More simple anatomical compression tends to lead to more accessible operative treatment.

2.3. Pronator Teres Muscle and Pronator Syndrome

Branches of the median nerve pass the pronator teres (PT), flexor digitorum superficialis (FDS), flexor carpi radialis (FCR), and palmaris longus (PL) before passing through the PT muscle (Figure 1) [24]. In most people, the median nerve passes between the humeral (superficial) and ulnar (deep) head of PT, the prevailing location of the PMNC; in some people the latter is missing, and the nerve passes only under the humeral head of the muscle. Rare variations of the nerve passing behind the ulnar head or through the humeral head of PT have been described [25]. Thickened tendinous bands, fibrous arches, and intramuscular bands can arise from the muscles [2,6,11,15–18,20,24–27]. Hypertrophy of the PT muscle might impact the compression [17,25].

Median nerve compression by the PT muscle was first reported by Seyffarth in 1951 [28]. He suggested using the term pronator syndrome (PS), which remains the most common term to describe PMNCs. By PS, most authors mean various combinations of symptoms that usually include proximal volar forearm pain at the region of the PT muscle, with varied median neuropathy such as weakness and sensory changes. Symptoms are typically provoked by strenuous repetitive activity such as forearm pronosupination.

2.4. Flexor Digitorum Superficialis Arch and Superficialis/Pronator Syndrome

After PT, the nerve courses between the muscles flexor digitorum profundus (FDP) and FDS. In up to 75% of forearms, the FDS muscle has a fibrous leading edge that can be tight while covering the median nerve and anterior interosseous nerve (AIN) (Figure 3) [2,11,15–

18,20,24,29]. Even elbow extension alone can cause median nerve and AIN compression at the FDS arch in certain forearms [29]. To further distinguish and specify the compressive point over the median nerve and the very close relation between FDS and PT, the term superficialis/pronator syndrome was recently proposed by Tang [30].

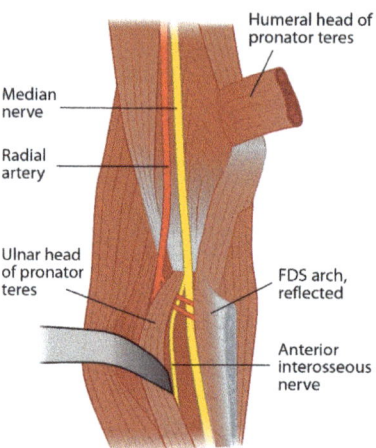

Figure 3. Leading tendinous edge of the flexor digitorum superficialis arch can cause compression of the median nerve and anterior interosseous nerve.

2.5. Anterior Interosseus Nerve and AIN Syndrome

AIN branches from the main median nerve at about the level of PT and innervates FDP2, flexor pollicis longus (FPL), and pronator quadratus (PQ). FDP3 is usually innervated by AIN but can be partially innervated by the ulnar nerve [31]. There are variations on the origin of AIN, however. When branching from the radial side of the median nerve, it is more susceptible to compression of musculoaponeurotic arches than when it originates from the posterior side [16]. A cadaveric study showed that AIN can easily be intraneurally separated from the main median nerve well above medial epicondyle level, even though the actual branching happens much more distally. The branch to the FCR arose from the AIN when dissected proximally [32]. In addition, in cases of trauma, oedema, or traction, small and less mobile nerves, such as AIN, have been shown to be at greater risk of injury and avulsions than bigger and more mobile nerves such as the main median nerve trunk [33–35].

Clearly differentiated from PS, anterior interosseous nerve syndrome (AINS) has been presented. Duchenne [36] reported one case of isolated palsy of the FPL already in 1872, but Kiloh and Nevin first described AINS in 1952 [37]. It is characterized by weakness or paralysis of FPL, FDP2, and PQ without sensory changes. Many authors discriminate an incomplete AIN palsy from a complete AIN palsy, and the term pseudo-AINS is also used for incomplete cases. It is debated whether AINS is a compression neuropathy or not.

2.6. Other Compressive Structures

On rare occasions, patients have been described to have other compression points, including vascular structures, thrombosis of crossing vessels, enlarged bicipital bursa, scar, hypertrophic brachialis muscle, and anomalous muscles surrounding the median nerve [11,15–17,20,38,39].

2.7. Distal Course of the Median Nerve

The palmar cutaneous branch of the median nerve (PCBMN) emerges about 5 cm proximal to the wrist crease. It usually runs between the tendons of FCR, and PL. PCBMN gives sensory branches to the skin at the palm and thenar area. Anatomical variations exist. The main median nerve then continues inside the carpal tunnel dividing into a motor branch to the thenar and a sensory branch to the thumb, index, long, and radial side of the ring finger.

2.8. Other Conflicting Factors

2.8.1. Martin–Gruber Anastomosis

Martin–Gruber anastomosis is an anomalous nerve connection from the median nerve to the ulnar nerve. It is prevalent in about 20% of the population [40]. Multiple branching variations have been described, but the two most common are from the main median nerve trunk before the pronator teres branch and from the AIN branch. Its significance appears in high ulnar nerve injuries when the normal median nerve can preserve a better distal sensory and motor function in the ulnar nerve distribution. Conversely, neuropathy in the median nerve can sometimes lead to symptoms in the ulnar part of the hand. Therefore, proximal median nerve compression can result in more diverse symptoms that would normally be expected [31,41].

2.8.2. Nerve Lesions and Renervation

Classifications for nerve injury have been described by Seddon [42] and Sunderland [43]. However, nerve injury can also be a mixture of the different grades and has a varying potential for recovery. Symptoms of momentary ischemia by external compression resolve quickly, but scarring by prolonged compression or axonal damage requires surgical decompression to enable nerve recovery. More difficult injury takes longer to heal and renervation speed is limited. Chronic denervation leads to permanent muscle fibrosis. Within these physiological boundaries, decisions must be made regarding the need for surgical intervention.

2.8.3. Double Crush Syndrome

Double crush syndrome was first hypothesized in 1973 by Upton and McComas [44]. Their clinical and electrodiagnostic observations led to the suspicion that one compression site of a nerve makes it more susceptible to other compressions. This clinical hypothesis was later confirmed in animal models and humans, as nerve compression leads to changes in axoplasmic flow and decreased transport of neurotrophic substances [45].

Distal median nerve compression, CTS, is more common than PMNC. Some patients with CTS experience pain also in the proximal arm and shoulder. In 1996, Lundborg suggested the term reverse double crush to reflect that a distal compression of a nerve predisposes it to proximal compressions and symptoms [46].

With the understanding of double or multiple crush syndromes, it has also been proposed that because there are many smaller potential sites of compression of the median nerve, all of which are asymptomatic by themselves, the cumulation of these compressions may eventually result in clinical problems for the patient. In addition, more general factors impairing the function of nerves, such as smoking, alcoholism, diabetes, and thyroid disease, are independent crushes themselves that need to be addressed [45].

2.8.4. Neuralgic Amyotrophy

In 1948, Parsonage and Turner reported an unusual syndrome of pain and paralysis around the shoulder in soldiers during the war years [47]. The name neuralgic amyotrophy (NA) was proposed, but named after the physicians, Parsonage–Turner syndrome has also been used for this condition. NA can be presented in multiple ways, but classically sudden pain at the top of the shoulder blade develops, lasting for a few days or weeks, eventually leading to paralysis of the shoulder girdle. Most patients with NA have difficulties in scapulothoracic movements, resulting in scapular winging, typically affecting the long thoracic and suprascapular nerves. Some patients develop median nerve sensory changes, and, like AINS, some patients also develop weakness of the AIN innervated muscles. The pathophysiology of NA remains unknown and likely includes genetic, autoimmune, and mechanical factors [48].

3. Clinical Presentation

3.1. Symptoms

Differential diagnosis for PMNC should include CTS but also nerve root compression at the cervical spine and compression at the brachial plexus such as TOS. Cervical radiculopathy usually causes more severe pain than PMNC and the pain radiates from the neck to the distal hand. TOS is a condition in which symptoms can consist of nerve, artery or vein compressions. However, due to variations in anatomy and multiple possible sites of compression, the symptoms vary across patients, and diagnosing TOS can be difficult.

The most common symptom in PMNC is pain at the proximal volar forearm, hand or fingers [2–4,15,17,19,26,49–51], sometimes radiating to the elbow, the axilla, and the head [52]. Patients may complain of aching discomfort, stiffening of the muscles in the forearm, cramping, clumsiness, loss of strength, and tonic flexion position of the fingers [15,17,28,51,52]. Flexion weakness of fingers can be wide-ranging or limited mostly to the AIN-innervated muscles FPL and FDP2 [23,53,54]. Symptoms typically begin insidiously but occasionally rapidly after muscle sprain or an episode of activity [15,17,19]. They might be work-related in various tasks ranging from writing or reading to heavy manual work with forceful forearm rotations and gripping, e.g., when using a screwdriver, carrying heavy objects or hammering [15,26–28,50,54]. Such sports as weight training, rowing, and racket games are possible predisposing factors [17,50,55]. In PMNC, symptoms are usually aggravated by activity but can resolve with rest and return when work resumes [28,50].

Many patients complain of numbness, tingling or sensory loss in the median nerve distribution area, sometimes in the palmar cutaneous branch of the median nerve [2–4,15,17, 26,28,49,51,56]. The difference between patients with PMNC and CTS is that with proximal compression patients usually do not experience the nocturnal awakening typically associated with CTS [2,17,26,50,52]. In addition, CTS does not cause paresthesias in the PCBMN. Both in a series of 343 patients with CTS and in another series with 101 patients, about 6% of patients were also diagnosed with PS [2,50]. In a third series, out of 146 patients who had undergone CTR, 13% were later diagnosed with PS [57].

The main symptom described in classic AINS is the partial or full disappearance of pinch grip between the thumb and index finger, usually unilaterally. Loss of PQ strength is more difficult to notice [58]. AIN is a motor nerve, so no sensory alterations occur. Prodromal pain in the shoulder, arm, or elbow may be present. The aetiologies of anatomical compression, physical exertion, repetitive activity, infection, vaccination, pregnancy, supracondylar humerus fracture on children, sleeping on an arm, forearm immobilization, and surgery unrelated to AIN (e.g., shoulder arthroscopy) have been described, but sometimes there is no apparent cause [18,33,35,59–65].

3.2. Clinical Findings

All possible median nerve compression sites should be examined, especially in the carpal tunnel, with tests such as Phalen's, Durkan's, or Tetro's test. Many patients have positive findings for PMNC and CTS simultaneously [17]. Concomitant ulnar nerve compression must be examined [66]. Thenar muscle tenderness can occur because of proximal problems in the median nerve [28]. In rare cases, muscle atrophy in the forearm can appear as well as atrophy of the thenar muscle [15].

All clinical tests for PMNC are subjective reports made by the examiner, which makes the diagnosis difficult and requires clinical experience. Because a troubled nerve has a lower threshold to withstand pressure, clinical tests that compress the nerve even more are designed to provoke patients' symptoms (Figure 4). Sensitivity and specificity of these tests have not been defined.

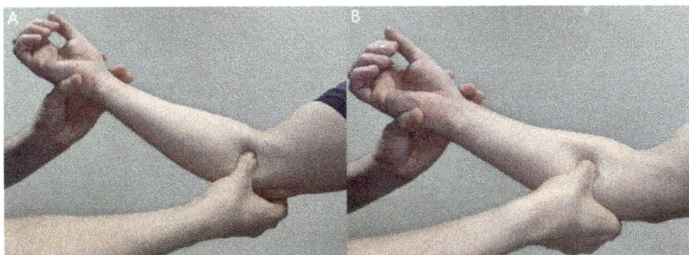

Figure 4. Manual compression of the median nerve at lacertus fibrosus (**A**) or at pronator teres and FDS arch (**B**) produces local pain and even distal paresthesia, indicating a nerve compression at that level. Compression test must also be performed at the Struthers' ligament proximal to the elbow joint level.

A classic finding in AINS is weakness or inability to make an "OK sign" due to dysfunction of FPL and FDP2 (Figure 5) [18,58–60]. However, patients with other PMNCs may present with this finding along with other muscle weaknesses [23,28,50]. In addition, AINS is sometimes mistaken for FPL tendon rupture [59].

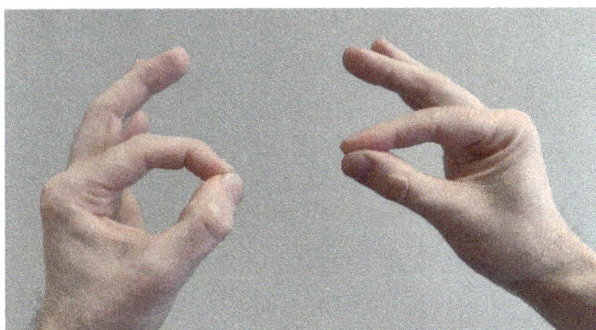

Figure 5. FPL and FDP2 weakness in the right hand and inability to make the OK sign indicates nerve injury proximal to the muscles mentioned.

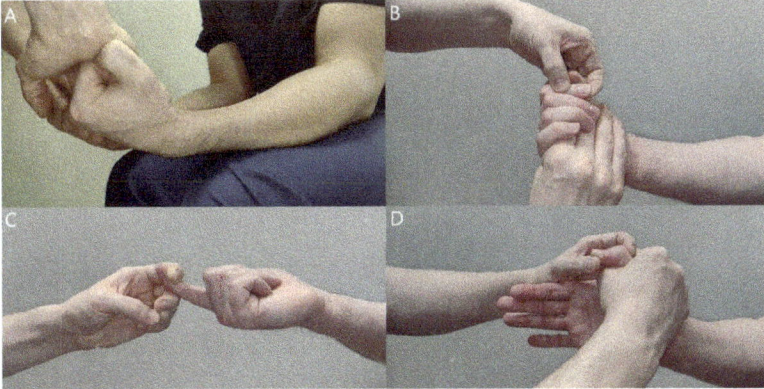

Figure 6. Resisted wrist (**A**), FDP2 (**B**,**C**), and FPL (**D**) flexion reveals minor weaknesses that the patient might not have yet registered. Weakness in the muscle indicates compression of the median nerve proximal to the site of muscle innervation. All tests must be compared with the unaffected side.

Patients with difficult aching pain in the forearm may only have minor muscle weaknesses. Careful, thorough muscle testing, compared with the unaffected side, is imperative to get a general perception of the neuropathy (Figures 5–9) [23,50,52].

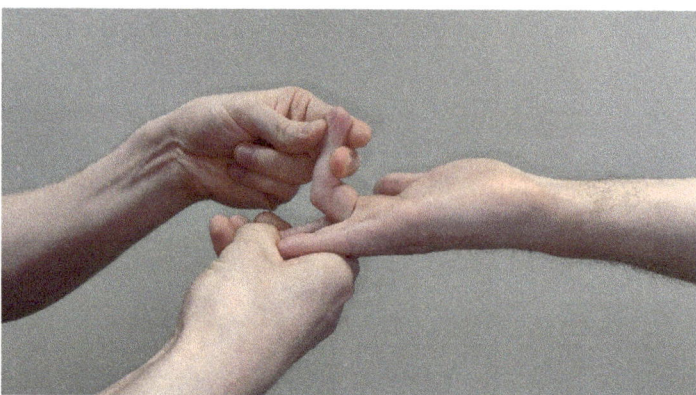

Figure 7. Resisted FDS3 flexion causes pain proximal in the forearm, indicating a nerve compression at the FDS arch.

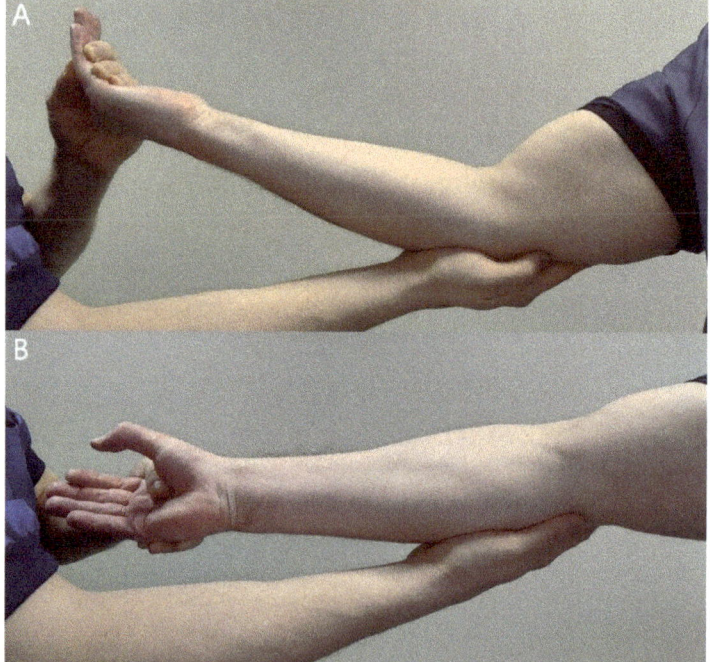

Figure 8. Resisted elbow flexion tightens the lacertus fibrosus and compresses the median nerve, causing local pain and sometimes distal paresthesia (**A**). Resisted forearm pronation in full supination tightens the pronator teres and compresses the median nerve (**B**). Local pain and a loss of pronation power can be observed compared with the unaffected side.

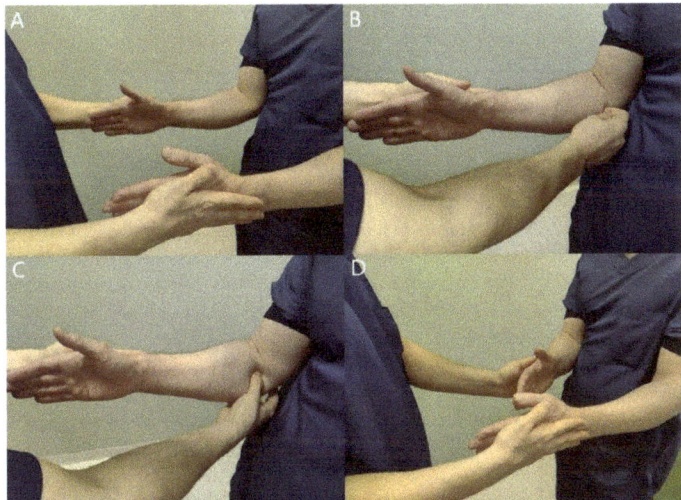

Figure 9. Scratch collapse test. With the patient's elbows flexed at 90 degrees and the arms held at the sides, the patient externally rotates the arms while the examiner resists the movement (**A**). After releasing the resistance of the rotation, the skin on top of the median nerve is scratched (**B**). Instead of scratching the skin, the examiner can compress the median nerve at the point of maximal tenderness (**C**). After the median nerve irritation, the patient is temporarily unable to resist the rotating force and the affected arm collapses, indicating a proximal compression of the nerve (**D**).

Along with symptom-provoking and muscle-weakness testing, sensory dysfunction must be explored. This can be done with tests for two-point discrimination or Semmes–Weinstein monofilaments from the median nerve innervated fingers and the PCBMN. As with muscle weakness, sensory deficits may be mild.

3.3. Electroneuromyography (ENMG)

Special expertise in performing ENMG in PMNC is needed. In PMNC, compression usually causes only occasional ischemia. Therefore, ENMG studies are neither efficient nor reliable in finding PMNC, especially in early symptoms, including pain and paresthesia. Severe clinical findings can only be seen at the late stages of neuropathy [67]. Most studies of PMNC report positive ENMG findings in a minority of patients [1–4,17,27,51,52,57,68]. However, studies reporting ENMG findings in the majority of patients probably represent more severe cases [15,69].

In patients with clinically diagnosed AIN weakness, ENMG findings are typically clearer but sometimes more wide-ranging than clinically expected, as complete or near-complete denervation can be seen in FPL, FDP2, and PQ [18,58,59,70]. The injury site can be more proximal than initially thought [61,68]. Repeated ENMG studies can track recovery.

3.4. Imaging Studies

Some authors suggest radiographs of the distal humerus, possibly revealing the supracondylar process and the possibility of a ligament of Struthers [12,13].

Ultrasound (US) evaluation of the nerve can be used to identify possible compression neuropathy and to assist perineural injections. Changes in nerve caliber and muscle perfusion can help to diagnose median nerve neuropathies if sufficiently severe [1,71–73].

In determining the aetiology of AINS, magnetic resonance imaging (MRI) might be useful to differentiate between NA and compression and to identify rare tumors in atypical cases [58,70,74,75]. Fascicular (or hourglass) constrictions of unknown origin, potentially trauma, inflammation, or autoimmune, are a common finding in recent imaging and surgical studies of AINS, suggesting neuritis such as NA. Interestingly, in MRI studies these fascicular constrictions can also locate at the upper arm level in median nerve fascicles that distally form the AIN branch [58,70]. Diagnostic imaging might not always be as helpful in decision-making as clinical evaluation in patients with other PMNCs. Of all patients with clinically diagnosed PS, 57% tested positive on US, and only 5% were positive on MRI [57].

4. Treatment

Literature on treatment of PMNC consists of heterogeneous hospital-based case series or reports without comparison of treatments. Most of the reports include surgery, but the extent of reporting the state of the nerve and whether thorough decompression of all possible sites of compression was performed varies across the studies. Due to the complexity of PMNCs, the accuracy of diagnoses can understandably be questioned.

4.1. Non-Operative Treament

A trial of conservative therapy with activity modifications is advisable. As the focus of management is on relieving pressure over the nerve, forearm pronosupination, gripping, flexing the elbow, and other strenuous repetitive activities should be diminished. Even total cessation of strenuous activity can be tried. Job modifications by changing elbow or forearm position during activity might be useful. Frequent breaks to supinate the forearm are encouraged if the patient works in front of the computer [17,28,50,55,76]. Good results have been reported for up to 70% of patients [28,50].

Injecting local anesthetics [28] or corticosteroids [50] to the PT muscle area has been reported. US-guided injection gave relief of symptoms to PS patients in one series [72].

In patients with AIN weakness, modification of upper and lower arm activity can be made as in other PMNCs. Different supportive treatments could be tried, but most studies report only waiting for spontaneous nerve recovery. In the absence of a clear cause or trauma, most patients with even total AIN palsy can be observed for spontaneous recovery, with good results [18,62]. Still, in up to 30% of patients, weakness or palsy remains [64].

4.2. Operative Treatment

Currently, no trials comparing operative and non-operative treatment exist, nor is there a consensus regarding the indications for operative treatment for PMNC. However, the general expert opinion is that surgical release is warranted in PMNC if symptoms are progressive or non-operative treatment is insufficient after a 3-month trial [15,61,62,66,69].

When operating on PMNC, all potential sites of pathology, including the ligament of Struthers, lacertus fibrosus, PT, and FDS arch, should be decompressed [17,51,55]. All fibrotic bands must be released along the course of the median nerve and AIN at the level of proximal forearm and distal arm if needed. PT fascia can be elongated to gain better exposure to the nerve. Afterwards, the compressive site of the nerve presents with the paucity of vasculature distally and increased tortuosity of the vasa nervorum proximally [51].

In a series of 27 patients with PMNC treated by Mackinnon, surgical decompression provided satisfactory outcomes for 93% of patients measured by improvements in strength, pain, quality of life, and DASH scores [51]. In a series of 55 surgically treated patients with PMNC, 80% reported good outcomes and 96% would undergo the operation again. Long progression time of symptoms significantly correlated with persisting symptoms at follow-up. In 51% of patients, the recovery was immediate, and in 49% it took more than 3 months [15]. Good results have been reported, with up to 90% of patients satisfied with the outcome [3,4,6,17,20,26,52,54].

A transverse incision [77] and an endoscopic technique [27,69] have been presented to minimize the length of the scar and to promote faster healing. In the study of Lee and colleagues [69], all 13 endoscopically operated patients received a significant improvement in DASH scores [69]. Still, a limited decompression might increase the risk of residual nerve impingement. With a small transverse incision in the forearm of 21 patients, the outcome for 12 (57%) was excellent or good, for 6 (29%) fair and for 3 (14 %) poor in the series reported by Tsai and colleagues [77]. With a careful clinical examination of the compressive site, many authors use a small incision with wide-awake local anesthesia without a tourniquet (WALANT) to treat LS, allowing perioperative testing of strength recovery after decompression of the nerve [22,23,30].

Patients with one clear mechanical cause or an apparent injury causing the symptoms seem to benefit from surgery the most. In a case series by Seitz and colleagues [19], all 7 patients with an acute injury to the elbow causing a partial rupture of biceps brachii, thus tethering the lacertus fibrosus over the median nerve, showed almost immediate relief of symptoms after surgery [19]. In 44 patients with compression under the lacertus fibrosus, Hagert [23] showed significant improvement after surgery; in most of them the improvement was immediate [23]. In addition, releasing the median nerve under the supracondylar process and the ligament of Struthers led to complete relief of symptoms in most patients compared with patients with more diffuse compression points [8,9,12–14].

The literature on surgery for AINS is limited to case reports or series that reveal an inconsistent benefit or varying recovery times. Hill and colleagues reported a series of 24 patients with surgically treated AINS; 8 of these patients returned to full function within 3 months or less, but the rest of them were slower to recover, taking up to 2 years [18]. Ulrich and colleagues noted that 13 out of 14 patients with AINS recovered well after surgery that was performed 12 weeks after initial symptoms [62]. In a case series by Park and colleagues, 11 patients with AINS treated conservatively for at least 6 months with no improvement were then surgically treated; a good outcome was recorded in 10 and a fair outcome in 1 patient [60]. In another series of 15 patients by Schantz, 9 patients improved at 7 weeks postoperatively [59]. Spinner reported full or partial recovery in just 3–12 weeks postoperatively [78]. Interestingly, Hill presented a patient with paralyzed FPL for 4 years who attained full function at 5 weeks after neurolysis [18].

If surgery is needed, a short immobilization with dressings or a splint for a few days after surgery followed by active mobilization is advised. After the wound has healed, a strengthening program is started. Return to work varies but return to sports is advised at 6 to 8 weeks after extensive surgery. Shorter wounds and smaller operations tend to lead to a much faster recovery, often in just a few days [23,27,69].

While adequate surgical management of PMNC usually gives satisfactory results, recurrence of symptoms has been described [17]. Even with multiple sites of compression of the median nerve in the forearm and carpal tunnel, initial management can resolve all the symptoms, at least temporarily. According to the literature on double crush syndrome, releasing one site of compression may revive the nerve for a while even if another remains unreleased, however, recurrence of symptoms is likely [45]. This might be the case with patients with suspected recurrence of CTS [17,79].

5. Discussion

CTS is widely diagnosed and treated. As PMNC symptoms can resemble CTS, these two conditions are often confused with each other. As a rarer diagnosis, PMNC might be underdiagnosed and left untreated. An undiagnosed PMNC might explain why all the patients with CTS do not recover after CTR [79]. In addition, due to Martin–Gruber anastomosis, symptoms of PMNC might mimic ulnar neuropathies. This can confuse diagnosing the condition but may also explain residual symptoms after properly executed ulnar nerve release.

CTS and PMNC can coexist in the same patient [2,17]. Olehnik and colleagues described their protocol for treating patients with symptoms of median nerve compression if the diagnosis was not certain for either CTS or PMNC. If ENMG is positive for CTS, they usually recommend only CTR, expecting some of the proximal symptoms to diminish as well. However, if ENMG is negative for CTS, they strongly advise proximal median nerve decompression as the initial procedure [4].

The variability of nerve injury needs to be understood. Compression neuropathies typically cause only mild changes such as neurapraxia or demyelination at most. When clinical findings are minor, PMNC is mostly a clinical diagnosis, and many criticize objective measurements, such as ENMG, to make the diagnosis [23,51]. However, axonopathy can occur in severe cases, which makes ENMG and other imaging studies necessary. In addition, poor recovery postoperatively could be due to residual impingement or more difficult initial nerve injury. The rate of nerve regeneration must be considered when progress is slow.

Whether nerve decompression surgery is beneficial compared with spontaneous recovery has been debated. When repetition and posture are related to onset of PMNC, the treatment should begin conservatively. Work modifications and reduction of strenuous activity can resolve symptoms by lessening muscle compressions over the nerve. Even nerve problems resulting from NA, inflammation, transient compression or trauma could spontaneously recover if the nerve is intact with no scarring. In most studies, if spontaneous recovery failed after a few months, surgery was performed. Due to a lack of randomized trials, the benefit of surgery relative to conservative treatment is unknown.

Treatment of AINS remains controversial due to difficulties in properly defining the cause. In their critical review on AINS, Krishnan and colleagues suggested that AINS is a form of NA and might not originate from compression in the forearm [64]. ENMG findings and imaging nerve fascicular contractions with MRI or US could provide clarification [70,71]. Without any evident compression over the nerve, normal regeneration might take place. With no spontaneous recovery, surgical decompression can be performed, preferably exploring the distal arm, and decompressing all encountered fascicular constrictions [41,64].

However, AINS can also be caused by compression. In a series of 44 patients with LS who benefitted greatly from surgical decompression, Hagert found that the most profound symptom was distinct weakness of muscles FPL, FDP2, and FCR. Only rarely did these patients have distal paresthesia [23]. In reports of AINS, FCR strength is seldom mentioned. AINS might sometimes be labelled too eagerly as neuritis, without a thorough clinical examination to identify a possible site of compression.

Because of potential multiple PMNC sites, some authors suggest separate names for the syndromes to distinguish them. The difference between LS and superficialis/pronator syndrome was discussed by Tang in a recent article suggesting the separation of these two [30]. Both Hagert and Tang encourage a selective mini-invasive technique for decompression with no need to release all potential compression sites. In turn, Sos and colleagues found no isolated compression over the AIN branch, but a compression proximal to it, in patients with classical AINS. They concluded that the proximal median nerve trunk must be explored even in patients without sensory symptoms and stated that there is no interest in distinguishing AINS from PS. Moreover, they criticized specific tests for nerve compression sites because they did not correlate with the actual entrapment sites found in surgery [15]. It is not uncommon to encounter two or more compressive structures over the median nerve in the surgery [3,17]. Mackinnon stated that it is impossible to reliably distinguish the compressive structures preoperatively and recommended a complete surgical release of the median nerve and AIN branch to minimize the risk of recurrence [51].

Tight lacertus fibrosus might cause pain, tightness, and swelling of the proximal flexor-pronator mass during repetitive forearm motion without apparent distal sensation symptoms, referring to an exertional compartment syndrome [80]. On the other hand, recent reviews of chronic exertional compartment syndrome of the forearm described patients characterized by pain in the volar forearm, decreased muscle strength, stiffness, and paresthesia in the fingers [81,82]. ENMG is negative, and patients benefit significantly from fasciotomies. The difference between PMNC and chronic exertional compartment syndrome in the forearm is therefore also questionable. The benefit of surgery could derive from fasciotomy but also from simultaneous nerve decompression.

This review presented available information of symptoms, diagnosis, treatment, and outcome of PMNC. Still, understanding of PMNC is far from complete. Good-quality clinical research is needed. Future research should focus on identifying the natural process and epidemiology of PMNC. The differential diagnosis between compression neuropathy and NA remains unclear. The cause of fascicular constrictions in AIN warrants closer investigations. More detailed information on certain symptoms and related clinical findings would be useful. Treatment guidelines rely on expert opinion and need to be properly addressed. Randomized trials are needed to clarify the need for surgery compared with conservative treatment.

6. Conclusions

Due to variability in anatomy and nerve injury, the findings in PMNC can range from subtle weakness to palsy and muscle atrophy. As clear objective signs do not always exist, PMNC is usually a clinical diagnosis with emphasis on tests that provoke symptoms and identify muscle weaknesses. This must be remembered when interpreting ENMG and imaging studies. Uncertainty about the etiology and treatment of AIN-related paresis remains, with some cases apparently caused by compression and others not. Sensory and motor symptoms of PMNC can mimic CTS, and this should be borne in mind, especially if CTR does not resolve all CTS symptoms in a patient.

A nerve injury regardless of etiology can recover spontaneously provided that the nerve remains intact, but pros and cons of surgery should be carefully and individually weighed if no recovery occurs. If needed, surgical decompression of all possible compression sites can yield satisfactory results.

In PMNC, several simultaneous compressive structures might exist that could go unnoticed with an overly limited view. Therefore, the need to separate PMNCs into smaller anatomy-based syndromes can be questioned, as none of them truly represent the mixture of overlapping anatomical variations encountered in clinical practice. Before clear progress in clinical research can be achieved, proximal median nerve-related pain and motor and sensory symptoms of multiple different etiologies should be named more comprehensively as a proximal median nerve syndrome.

Author Contributions: Conceptualization, P.L. and J.R.; methodology, P.L. and S.H.; investigation, P.L. and S.H.; writing—original draft preparation, P.L.; writing—review and editing, P.L., S.H. and J.R.; visualization, P.L.; supervision, J.R. All authors have read and agreed to the published version of the manuscript.

Funding: Seinäjoki Central Hospital funded the journal's open access and article processing charge (APC). This research was funded by a Finnish Medical Foundation grant for S.H. (Grant number 5302).

Institutional Review Board Statement: Not applicable.

Informed Consent Statement: Not applicable.

Data Availability Statement: Not applicable.

Conflicts of Interest: The authors declare no conflict of interest.

References

1. Asheghan, M.; Hollisaz, M.T.; Aghdam, A.S.; Khatibiaghda, A. The Prevalence of Pronator Teres among Patients with Carpal Tunnel Syndrome: Cross-Sectional Study. *Int. J. Biomed. Sci.* **2016**, *12*, 89–94. [PubMed]
2. Hsiao, C.-W.; Shih, J.-T.; Hung, S.-T. Concurrent Carpal Tunnel Syndrome and Pronator Syndrome: A Retrospective Study of 21 Cases. *Orthop. Traumatol. Surg. Res.* **2017**, *103*, 101–103. [CrossRef] [PubMed]
3. Mujadzic, M.; Papanicolaou, G.; Young, H.; Tsai, T.-M. Simultaneous Surgical Release of Ipsilateral Pronator Teres and Carpal Tunnel Syndromes. *Plast. Reconstr. Surg.* **2007**, *119*, 2141–2147. [CrossRef] [PubMed]
4. Olehnik, W.K.; Manske, P.R.; Szerzinski, J. Median Nerve Compression in the Proximal Forearm. *J. Hand Surg. Am.* **1994**, *19*, 121–126. [CrossRef]
5. Luangjarmekorn, P.; Tsai, T.M.; Honsawek, S.; Kitidumrongsook, P. Role of Pronator Release in Revision Carpal Tunnel Surgery. *SICOT J.* **2016**, *2*, 9. [CrossRef]
6. Gainor, B.J. The Pronator Compression Test Revisited. A Forgotten Physical Sign. *Orthop. Rev.* **1990**, *19*, 888–892.
7. Struthers, J. On a Peculiarity of the Humerus and Humeral Artery. *Mon. J. Med. Sci.* **1848**, *28*, 264–267. [CrossRef]
8. Ivins, G.K. Supracondylar Process Syndrome: A Case Report. *J. Hand Surg. Am.* **1996**, *21*, 279–281. [CrossRef]

9. Kessel, L.; Rang, M. Supracondylar Spur of the Humerus. *J. Bone Jt. Surg. Br.* **1966**, *48*, 765–769. [CrossRef]
10. Barnard, L.B.; McCoy, S.M. The Supra Condyloid Process of the Humerus. *J. Bone Jt. Surg. Am.* **1946**, *28*, 845–850.
11. Bilecenoglu, B.; Uz, A.; Karalezli, N. Possible Anatomic Structures Causing Entrapment Neuropathies of the Median Nerve: An Anatomic Study. *Acta Orthop. Belg.* **2005**, *71*, 169–176. [PubMed]
12. Shon, H.-C.; Park, J.-K.; Kim, D.-S.; Kang, S.-W.; Kim, K.-J.; Hong, S.-H. Supracondylar Process Syndrome: Two Cases of Median Nerve Neuropathy Due to Compression by the Ligament of Struthers. *J. Pain Res.* **2018**, *11*, 803–807. [CrossRef] [PubMed]
13. Opanova, M.I.; Atkinson, R.E. Supracondylar Process Syndrome: Case Report and Literature Review. *J. Hand Surg. Am.* **2014**, *39*, 1130–1135. [CrossRef]
14. Gessini, L.; Jandolo, B.; Pietrangeli, A. Entrapment Neuropathies of the Median Nerve at and above the Elbow. *Surg. Neurol.* **1983**, *19*, 112–116. [CrossRef]
15. Sos, C.; Roulet, S.; Lafon, L.; Corcia, P.; Laulan, J.; Bacle, G. Median Nerve Entrapment Syndrome in the Elbow and Proximal Forearm. Anatomic Causes and Results for a 55-Case Surgical Series at a Mean 7years' Follow-Up. *Orthop. Traumatol. Surg. Res.* **2021**, *107*, 102825. [CrossRef]
16. Dellon, A.L.; Mackinnon, S.E. Musculoaponeurotic Variations along the Course of the Median Nerve in the Proximal Forearm. *J. Hand Surg. Br.* **1987**, *12*, 359–363. [CrossRef]
17. Hartz, C.R.; Linscheid, R.L.; Gramse, R.R.; Daube, J.R. The Pronator Teres Syndrome: Compressive Neuropathy of the Median Nerve. *J. Bone Jt. Surg. Am.* **1981**, *63*, 885–890. [CrossRef]
18. Hill, N.A.; Howard, F.M.; Huffer, B.R. The Incomplete Anterior Interosseous Nerve Syndrome. *J. Hand Surg. Am.* **1985**, *10*, 4–16. [CrossRef]
19. Seitz, W.H.; Matsuoka, H.; McAdoo, J.; Sherman, G.; Stickney, D.P. Acute Compression of the Median Nerve at the Elbow by the Lacertus Fibrosus. *J. Shoulder Elb. Surg.* **2007**, *16*, 91–94. [CrossRef]
20. Matsuzaki, A. Operative Treatment of Pronator Syndrome. *Orthop. Traumatol.* **1999**, *7*, 34–43. [CrossRef]
21. Bennett, G.E. Injuries Characteristic of Particular Sports Elbow and Shoulder Lesions of Baseball Players. *Am. J. Surg.* **1959**, *98*, 484–492. [CrossRef]
22. Hagert, E.; Lalonde, D.H. Lacertus Syndrome: Median Nerve Release at the Elbow. In *Wide Awake Hand Surgery*; Lalonde, D.H., Ed.; Thieme: New York, NY, USA, 2016; pp. 141–145.
23. Hagert, E. Clinical Diagnosis and Wide-Awake Surgical Treatment of Proximal Median Nerve Entrapment at the Elbow: A Prospective Study. *HAND* **2013**, *8*, 41–46. [CrossRef] [PubMed]
24. Fuss, F.K.; Wurzl, G.H. Median Nerve Entrapment. Pronator Teres Syndrome. Surgical Anatomy and Correlation with Symptom Patterns. *Surg. Radiol. Anat.* **1990**, *12*, 267–271. [CrossRef] [PubMed]
25. Beaton, L.E.; Anson, B.J. The Relation of the Median Nerve to the Pronator Teres Muscle. Contribution no. 289 from the Anatomical Laboratories of Northwestern University Medical School. *Anat. Rec.* **1939**, *75*, 23–26. [CrossRef]
26. Werner, C.O.; Rosén, I.; Thorngren, K.G. Clinical and Neurophysiologic Characteristics of the Pronator Syndrome. *Clin. Orthop. Relat. Res.* **1985**, *197*, 231–236. [CrossRef]
27. Zancolli, E.R.; Zancolli, E.P.; Perrotto, C.J. New Mini-Invasive Decompression for Pronator Teres Syndrome. *J. Hand Surg. Am.* **2012**, *37*, 1706–1710. [CrossRef]
28. Seyffarth, H. Primary Myoses in the M. Pronator Teres as Cause of Lesion of the N. Medianus (the Pronator Syndrome). *Acta Psychiatr. Neurol. Scand. Suppl.* **1951**, *74*, 251–254.
29. Tubbs, R.S.; Marshall, T.; Loukas, M.; Shoja, M.M.; Cohen-Gadol, A.A. The Sublime Bridge: Anatomy and Implications in Median Nerve Entrapment. *J. Neurosurg.* **2010**, *113*, 110–112. [CrossRef]
30. Tang, J.B. Median Nerve Compression: Lacertus Syndrome versus Superficialis-Pronator Syndrome. *J. Hand. Surg. Eur. Vol.* **2021**, *46*, 1017–1022. [CrossRef]
31. Spinner, M.; Spencer, P.S. Nerve Compression Lesions of the Upper Extremity. A Clinical and Experimental Review. *Clin. Orthop. Relat. Res.* **1974**, *104*, 46–67. [CrossRef]
32. Jabaley, M.E.; Wallace, W.H.; Heckler, F.R. Internal Topography of Major Nerves of the Forearm and Hand: A Current View. *J. Hand Surg. Am.* **1980**, *5*, 1–18. [CrossRef]
33. Collins, D.N.; Weber, E.R. Anterior Interosseous Nerve Avulsion. *Clin. Orthop. Relat. Res.* **1983**, *181*, 175–178. [CrossRef]
34. Howard, F.M. Compression Neuropathies in the Anterior Forearm. *Hand Clin.* **1986**, *2*, 737–745. [CrossRef]
35. Vincelet, Y.; Journeau, P.; Popkov, D.; Haumont, T.; Lascombes, P. The Anatomical Basis for Anterior Interosseous Nerve Palsy Secondary to Supracondylar Humerus Fractures in Children. *Orthop. Traumatol. Surg. Res.* **2013**, *99*, 543–547. [CrossRef] [PubMed]
36. Duchenne de Boulogne, G.-B.-A. *De L'électrisation Localisée et de Son Application À La Pathologie et À La Thérapeutique*, 3rd ed.; Baillière, J.B., Ed.; J.-B. Baillière et Fils: Paris, France, 1872.
37. Kiloh, L.G.; Nevin, S. Isolated Neuritis of the Anterior Interosseous Nerve. *Br. Med. J.* **1952**, *1*, 850–851. [CrossRef]
38. Al-Qattan, M.M. Gantzer's Muscle. An Anatomical Study of the Accessory Head of the Flexor Pollicis Longus Muscle. *J. Hand Surg. Br.* **1996**, *21*, 269–270. [CrossRef]
39. Caetano, E.B.; Sabongi, J.J.; Vieira, L.Â.; Caetano, M.F.; Moraes, D.V. Gantzer Muscle. An Anatomical Study. *Acta Ortop. Bras.* **2015**, *23*, 72–75. [CrossRef]
40. Roy, J.; Henry, B.M.; Pękala, P.A.; Vikse, J.; Saganiak, K.; Walocha, J.A.; Tomaszewski, K.A. Median and Ulnar Nerve Anastomoses in the Upper Limb: A Meta-Analysis. *Muscle Nerve* **2016**, *54*, 36–47. [CrossRef]

41. Haussmann, P.; Patel, M.R. Intraepineurial Constriction of Nerve Fascicles in Pronator Syndrome and Anterior Interosseous Nerve Syndrome. *Orthop. Clin. N. Am.* **1996**, *27*, 339–344. [CrossRef]
42. Seddon, H.J. A Classification of Nerve Injuries. *Br. Med. J.* **1942**, *2*, 237–239. [CrossRef]
43. Sunderland, S. A Classification of Peripheral Nerve Injuries Producing Loss of Function. *Brain* **1951**, *74*, 491–516. [CrossRef] [PubMed]
44. Upton, A.R.; McComas, A.J. The Double Crush in Nerve Entrapment Syndromes. *Lancet* **1973**, *2*, 359–362. [CrossRef]
45. Mackinnon, S.E. Double and Multiple "Crush" Syndromes. Double and Multiple Entrapment Neuropathies. *Hand Clin.* **1992**, *8*, 369–390. [CrossRef]
46. Lundborg, G.; Dahlin, L.B. Anatomy, Function, and Pathophysiology of Peripheral Nerves and Nerve Compression. *Hand Clin.* **1996**, *12*, 185–193. [CrossRef]
47. Parsonege, M.J.; Turner, J.W.A. Neuralgic Amyotrophy; the Shoulder-Girdle Syndrome. *Lancet* **1948**, *1*, 973–978. [CrossRef]
48. van Eijk, J.J.J.; Groothuis, J.T.; van Alfen, N. Neuralgic Amyotrophy: An Update on Diagnosis, Pathophysiology, and Treatment. *Muscle Nerve* **2016**, *53*, 337–350. [CrossRef]
49. Lee, M.J.; LaStayo, P.C. Pronator Syndrome and Other Nerve Compressions That Mimic Carpal Tunnel Syndrome. *J. Orthop. Sports Phys. Ther.* **2004**, *34*, 601–609. [CrossRef]
50. Morris, H.H.; Peters, B.H. Pronator Syndrome: Clinical and Electrophysiological Features in Seven Cases. *J. Neurol. Neurosurg. Psychiatry* **1976**, *39*, 461–464. [CrossRef]
51. El-Haj, M.; Ding, W.; Sharma, K.; Novak, C.; Mackinnon, S.E.; Patterson, J.M.M. Median Nerve Compression in the Forearm: A Clinical Diagnosis. *Hand* **2021**, *16*, 586–591. [CrossRef]
52. Johnson, R.K.; Spinner, M.; Shrewsbury, M.M. Median Nerve Entrapment Syndrome in the Proximal Forearm. *J. Hand Surg. Am.* **1979**, *4*, 48–51. [CrossRef]
53. Lalonde, D. Minimally Invasive Anesthesia in Wide Awake Hand Surgery. *Hand Clin.* **2014**, *30*, 1–6. [CrossRef] [PubMed]
54. Stål, M.; Hagert, C.G.; Moritz, U. Upper Extremity Nerve Involvement in Swedish Female Machine Milkers. *Am. J. Ind. Med.* **1998**, *33*, 551–559. [CrossRef]
55. Mccue, F.C.I.; Alexander, E.J.; Baumgarten, T.E. Median Nerve Entrapment at the Elbow in Athletes. *Oper. Tech. Sports Med.* **1996**, *4*, 21–27. [CrossRef]
56. Gross, P.T.; Tolomeo, E.A. Proximal Median Neuropathies. *Neurol. Clin.* **1999**, *17*, 425–445. [CrossRef]
57. Özdemir, A.; Acar, M.A.; Güleç, A.; Durgut, F.; Cebeci, H. Clinical, Radiological, and Electrodiagnostic Diagnosis of Pronator Syndrome Concurrent With Carpal Tunnel Syndrome. *J. Hand Surg. Am.* **2020**, *45*, 1141–1147. [CrossRef]
58. Sneag, D.B.; Arányi, Z.; Zusstone, E.M.; Feinberg, J.H.; Queler, S.C.; Nwawka, O.K.; Lee, S.K.; Wolfe, S.W. Fascicular Constrictions above Elbow Typify Anterior Interosseous Nerve Syndrome. *Muscle Nerve* **2020**, *61*, 301–310. [CrossRef]
59. Schantz, K.; Riegels-Nielsen, P. The Anterior Interosseous Nerve Syndrome. *J. Hand Surg. Br.* **1992**, *17*, 510–512. [CrossRef]
60. Park, I.-J.; Roh, Y.-T.; Jeong, C.; Kim, H.-M. Spontaneous Anterior Interosseous Nerve Syndrome: Clinical Analysis of Eleven Surgical Cases. *J. Plast. Surg. Hand Surg.* **2013**, *47*, 519–523. [CrossRef] [PubMed]
61. Na, K.-T.; Jang, D.-H.; Lee, Y.-M.; Park, I.-J.; Lee, H.-W.; Lee, S.-U. Anterior Interosseous Nerve Syndrome: Is It a Compressive Neuropathy? *Indian J. Orthop.* **2020**, *54*, 193–198. [CrossRef]
62. Ulrich, D.; Piatkowski, A.; Pallua, N. Anterior Interosseous Nerve Syndrome: Retrospective Analysis of 14 Patients. *Arch. Orthop. Trauma. Surg.* **2011**, *131*, 1561–1565. [CrossRef]
63. Nammour, M.; Desai, B.; Warren, M.; Sisco-Wise, L. Anterior Interosseous Nerve Palsy After Shoulder Arthroscopy Treated With Surgical Decompression: A Case Series and Systematic Review of the Literature. *Hand* **2021**, *16*, 201–209. [CrossRef] [PubMed]
64. Krishnan, K.R.; Sneag, D.B.; Feinberg, J.H.; Wolfe, S.W. Anterior Interosseous Nerve Syndrome Reconsidered: A Critical Analysis Review. *JBJS Rev.* **2020**, *8*, e2000011. [CrossRef] [PubMed]
65. Joist, A.; Joosten, U.; Wetterkamp, D.; Neuber, M.; Probst, A.; Rieger, H. Anterior Interosseous Nerve Compression after Supracondylar Fracture of the Humerus: A Metaanalysis. *J. Neurosurg.* **1999**, *90*, 1053–1056. [CrossRef] [PubMed]
66. Skouteris, D.; Thoma, S.; Andritsos, G.; Tasios, N.; Praxitelous, P.; Psychoyios, V. Simultaneous Compression of the Median and Ulnar Nerve at the Elbow: A Retrospective Study. *J. Hand Surg. Asian Pac. Vol.* **2018**, *23*, 198–204. [CrossRef] [PubMed]
67. Tapadia, M.; Mozaffar, T.; Gupta, R. Compressive Neuropathies of the Upper Extremity: Update on Pathophysiology, Classification, and Electrodiagnostic Findings. *J. Hand Surg. Am.* **2010**, *35*, 668–677. [CrossRef] [PubMed]
68. Gross, P.T.; Jones, H.R. Proximal Median Neuropathies: Electromyographic and Clinical Correlation. *Muscle Nerve* **1992**, *15*, 390–395. [CrossRef]
69. Lee, A.K.; Khorsandi, M.; Nurbhai, N.; Dang, J.; Fitzmaurice, M.; Herron, K.A. Endoscopically Assisted Decompression for Pronator Syndrome. *J. Hand Surg. Am.* **2012**, *37*, 1173–1179. [CrossRef]
70. Pham, M.; Bäumer, P.; Meinck, H.-M.; Schiefer, J.; Weiler, M.; Bendszus, M.; Kele, H. Anterior Interosseous Nerve Syndrome: Fascicular Motor Lesions of Median Nerve Trunk. *Neurology* **2014**, *82*, 598–606. [CrossRef]
71. Hide, I.G.; Grainger, A.J.; Naisby, G.P.; Campbell, R.S. Sonographic Findings in the Anterior Interosseous Nerve Syndrome. *J. Clin. Ultrasound* **1999**, *27*, 459–464. [CrossRef]
72. Delzell, P.B.; Patel, M. Ultrasound-Guided Perineural Injection for Pronator Syndrome Caused by Median Nerve Entrapment. *J. Ultrasound Med.* **2020**, *39*, 1023–1029. [CrossRef]

73. Youngner, J.M.; Matsuo, K.; Grant, T.; Garg, A.; Samet, J.; Omar, I.M. Sonographic Evaluation of Uncommonly Assessed Upper Extremity Peripheral Nerves: Anatomy, Technique, and Clinical Syndromes. *Skelet. Radiol* **2019**, *48*, 57–74. [CrossRef] [PubMed]
74. Akman, Y.E.; Yalcinkaya, M.; Arikan, Y.; Kabukcuoglu, Y. Atypically Localized Glomus Tumor Causing Anterior Interosseous Nerve Syndrome: A Case Report. *Acta Orthop. Traumatol. Turc.* **2017**, *51*, 492–494. [CrossRef] [PubMed]
75. Afshar, A. Pronator Syndrome Due to Schwannoma. *J. Hand Microsurg.* **2015**, *7*, 119–122. [CrossRef] [PubMed]
76. Mackinnon, S.E.; Novak, C.B. Clinical Commentary: Pathogenesis of Cumulative Trauma Disorder. *J. Hand Surg. Am.* **1994**, *19*, 873–883. [CrossRef]
77. Tsai, T.M.; Syed, S.A. A Transverse Skin Incision Approach for Decompression of Pronator Teres Syndrome. *J. Hand Surg. Br.* **1994**, *19*, 40–42. [CrossRef]
78. Spinner, M. The Anterior Interosseous-Nerve Syndrome, with Special Attention to Its Variations. *J. Bone Jt. Surg. Am.* **1970**, *52*, 84–94. [CrossRef]
79. Hagert, E.; Curtis, C. Failed Carpal Tunnel Release: Recognizing the Lacertus Syndrome. In *Problems in Hand Surgery: Solutions to Recover Function*; Neumeister, M.W., Ed.; Thieme: New York, NY, USA, 2020; ISBN 9781626237094.
80. Jordan, S.E. The Lacertus Syndrome of the Elbow in Throwing Athletes. *Clin. Sports Med.* **2020**, *39*, 589–596. [CrossRef]
81. Willick, S.E.; Deluigi, A.J.; Taskaynatan, M.; Petron, D.J.; Coleman, D. Bilateral Chronic Exertional Compartment Syndrome of the Forearm: A Case Report and Review of the Literature. *Curr. Sports Med. Rep.* **2013**, *12*, 170–174. [CrossRef]
82. Smeraglia, F.; Tamborini, F.; Garutti, L.; Minini, A.; Basso, M.A.; Cherubino, M. Chronic Exertional Compartment Syndrome of the Forearm: A Systematic Review. *EFORT Open Rev.* **2021**, *6*, 101–106. [CrossRef]

Review

Optimization of Carpal Tunnel Syndrome Using WALANT Method

Kathryn R. Segal, Alexandria Debasitis and Steven M. Koehler *

Department of Orthopaedic Surgery, Albert Einstein College of Medicine, Montefiore Medical Center, Bronx, NY 10461, USA; kathryn.segal@einsteinmed.edu (K.R.S.); alexandria.debasitis@einsteinmed.edu (A.D.)
* Correspondence: stkoehler@montefiore.org

Abstract: As surgical management of carpal tunnel release (CTR) becomes ever more common, extensive research has emerged to optimize the contextualization of this procedure. In particular, CTR under the wide-awake, local-anesthesia, no-tourniquet (WALANT) technique has emerged as a cost-effective, safe, and straightforward option for the millions who undergo this procedure worldwide. CTR under WALANT is associated with considerable cost savings and workflow efficiencies; it can be safely and effectively executed in an outpatient clinic under field sterility with less use of resources and production of waste, and it has consistently demonstrated standard or better post-operative pain control and satisfaction among patients. In this review of the literature, we describe the current findings on CTR using the WALANT technique.

Keywords: carpal tunnel syndrome; carpal tunnel release; wide-awake anesthesia; local anesthesia; WALANT

1. Introduction

As the most common peripheral-nerve entrapment disorder worldwide, millions of individuals are affected by carpal tunnel syndrome (CTS) each year [1–4]. CTS has a wide variety of risk factors, including demographic (female sex), occupational (repetitive tasks and postures), and medical (obesity, pregnancy, renal failure, hypothyroidism, congenital heart failure, and distal radius fractures) [5]. Interestingly, Kasielska-Trojan et al. have even suggested a role for pre- and post-natal sex steroids in the development of CTS, which could explain the notably higher prevalence of CTS in the female population [6].

Meanwhile, surgical management through carpal tunnel release (CTR) has continued to increase in popularity and prevalence [7,8]. With this trend, there has been extensive research to contextualize the settings and conditions that optimize CTR. Wide-awake, local-anesthesia, no-tourniquet (WALANT) surgery has emerged as a feasible, safe and cost-effective option for a wide array of surgical procedures involving the hand, including CTR. In a 2020 survey of American hand surgeons, nearly 80% reported having performed WALANT surgeries during their career and over 60% were currently using WALANT in their practices [9]. Since that time, its popularity and utility has continued to grow, most notably during the recent COVID-19 pandemic where its feasibility in outpatient settings and its better infectious-safety profile resulting from the avoidance of aerosol-generating anesthesia were preferred [10,11].

In this review of the literature, we describe the current findings relating to the use of WALANT for CTR, particularly as it pertains to cost and efficiency, operative set-up and resource optimization, complications and safety, patient satisfaction and perspectives, pain control, and return to functioning. We also discuss contraindications to the use of WALANT.

2. Efficiencies and Cost Savings

Efficiencies and cost savings have long been established with WALANT procedures, including CTR. Studies that have looked at these issues have particularly focused on: savings associated with clinic-based surgery; peri-operative metrics such as total procedural time; direct costs between CTR under WALANT and other types of anesthesia; and its scalability and applicability in low-resource settings. Additionally, considerable cost savings have been achieved from optimizing the room set-up and instruments used, which we discuss in greater detail in the next section.

2.1. Clinic-Based Procedures

It is becoming more common for CTR to be performed in outpatient clinics [12]. As such, considerable cost savings have been derived from integrating CTR into this less costly setting. Leblanc et al. originally estimated that the cost of CTR performed in an ambulatory setting was close to one-fourth of the cost of CTR performed in an operating room [13]. Similarly, Kazmers et al. found that a decrease in costs of an order greater than six-fold was associated with the performance of open CTR, under WALANT, in the clinic instead of in the traditional operating room. White et al. demonstrated average savings of nearly USD 400 at their institution when CTR was performed in the clinic instead of in an ambulatory surgery center (USD 151.92 versus USD 557.07, respectively) [14,15]. In addition to finding considerable cost savings with clinic-based CTR, Chatterjee et al. calculated an opportunity cost of USD 2700 when CTR was performed in an operating room instead of a clinic [16]. Moreover, Rogers et al. demonstrated through econometric modeling that office-based CTR not only achieves cost savings for the individuals involved, but results in significant cost reductions for the larger health care system and society as a whole [17].

2.2. Time Savings and Workflow Efficiencies

Several studies have also measured the time saved when CTR is performed under WALANT. When compared with IV anesthesia and sedation, Okamura et al. found that patients spent more time in the operating room, averaging an additional 13.5 min, when IV anesthesia was used. Alter et al. and Via et al. found significant time savings for WALANT patients, measured as the time spent in the post-anesthesia care unit (PACU) (average savings of 77 and 22 min, respectively, for the two procedures) [18–20]. Patients were able to leave the PACU more promptly following surgery under WALANT. Kamal et al. created a clinical pathway specific to CTR under WALANT that involved particular interventions such as: the administration of local anesthesia in a pre-operative holding room; a CTR-specific surgical tray; and prompt attention in the PACU. Following implementation of this pathway, the authors demonstrated a 31% reduction in total costs and 34% reduction in total time spent by patients at the facility, with no changes in quality of outcomes or patient experience [21]. Other studies have also demonstrated greater operative throughput and workflow efficiencies with the incorporation of WALANT [15,22].

In addition, WALANT has reduced the need for historically-based pre-operative assessments such as standard blood work, electrocardiograms, and chest radiographs. This allows patients to undergo CTR more promptly and seamlessly [23].

2.3. Estimates of Cost Savings

Several studies have estimated the direct cost savings associated with the use of CTR under WALANT. One single-center, single-surgeon study found that the total costs of CTR under WALANT amounted to USD 89.12 compared with USD 1409.28 for intravenous (IV) anesthesia [19]. When introducing hand surgery procedures under WALANT, 34% of which were CTR, a military medical center reported it saved USD 393,100 over a 21-month period [24]. One study found absolute cost savings of USD 390 from anesthesia services alone when performing CTR under WALANT, but the total costs were similar when controlled for the location of the clinical setting [20]. This finding suggests that the majority of cost savings achieved with WALANT are derived from setting-specific circumstances.

2.4. Scalability and Utilization in Low-Resource Settings

Barriers to surgical care and accessibility in low-resource regions have long been studied by the academic community [25]. The World Health Organization's Global Health Estimate suggested there was an unmet need for over 40 million musculoskeletal-related surgeries in calendar year 2010 [26]. In this context, use of WALANT with its considerable cost savings and lower utilization of resources provides an opportunity for drastic improvements in scalability and application in under-served regions. Though not studied for CTR specifically, Behar et al. and Holoyda et al. have described the successful integration of WALANT into a variety of hand procedures in clinics and in a teaching hospital in Kumasi, Ghana [27,28].

3. Operative Set-Up and Resource Optimization

As discussed, it has become increasingly popular for CTR, particularly under WALANT, to take place in the outpatient clinic. With this trend, it is important to consider how the procedure room differs from the traditional operating room. First, the use of field sterility instead of main-operating-room sterility has allowed for considerable cost and waste reductions, without impacting upon the likelihood of surgical site infections (Figure 1) [29–31]. Instead of needing the full standard set-up for main-operating-room sterility (which includes head covers, neck-to-knee sterile surgeon gowns, shoe covers, laminar airflow, and full-patient-body sterile draping), CTR can safely be performed in a clinic's procedure room with nothing more than a mask, sterile gloves, and single drape. Importantly, where CTR is performed in such settings, the absence of costly, specialized ventilation systems such as laminar air filtration or high-efficiency particulate air filters has not been linked to worse outcomes. Currently, more than 90% of CTRs by Canadian surgeons are performed under this minimalistic sterility set-up [32].

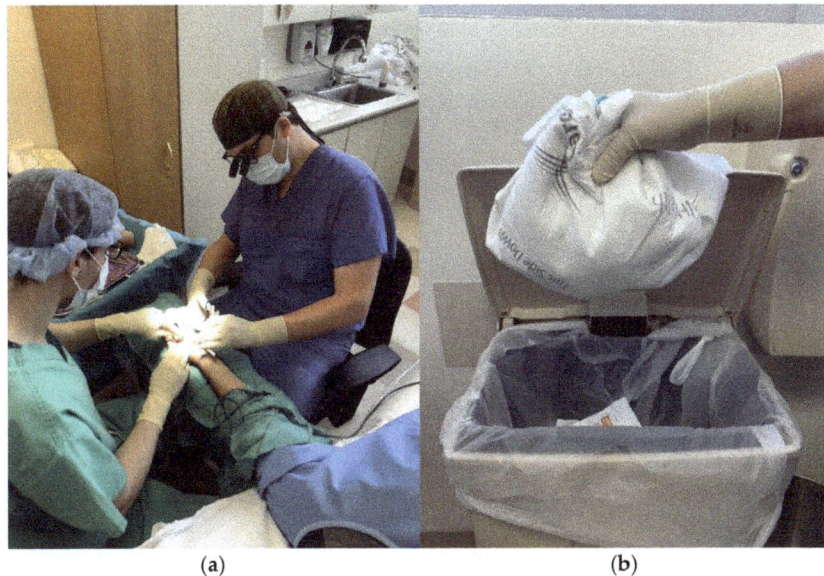

Figure 1. (**a**) Intraoperative set-up. Main surgical attending (**right**) is accompanied by a resident surgeon (**left**) during CTR under WALANT using field sterility. (**b**) Collection of all disposable materials from one CTR procedure.

Moreover, with a less complex room set-up, fewer personnel and surgical instruments are needed for successful execution of CTR. Avoricani et al. showed that hand surgeries under WALANT can safely be undertaken with a single circulating nurse instead of the two that are typically required by most institutions. Leblanc et al. showed that a considerable proportion of Canadian surgeons performed CTR without an anesthesia specialist present [13,33]. Kamal et al., in their clinical pathway for CTR under WALANT, describe creating an instrument pack specific to the CTR procedure to optimize workflow and reduce waste [21]. Maliha et al. found that the use of a surgery-specific instrument tray for trigger-finger release resulted in a 70% decrease in costs when compared with the standard instrument tray used in a traditional operating room [34]. This has been equally studied with regard to its applicability to WALANT. While not studied specifically for CTR, it is reasonable to assume that CTR-specific instrument trays also result in significant cost reductions and workflow efficiencies. The layout and contents of CTR-specific surgical tables and instrument trays are shown in Figure 2.

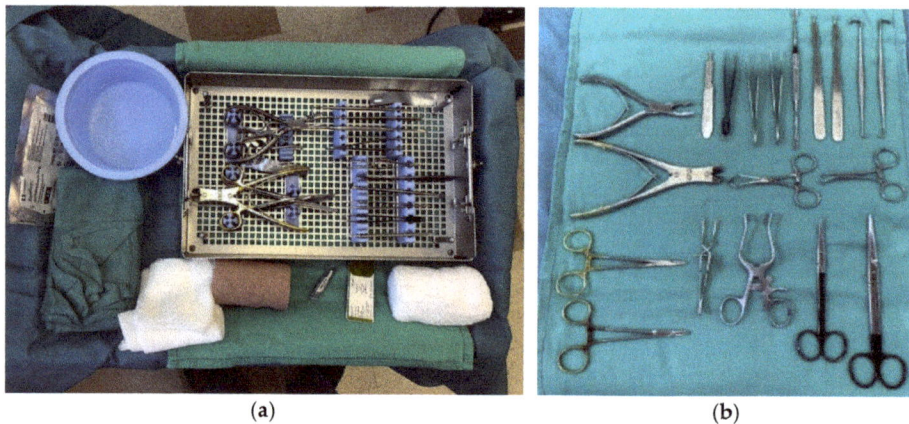

Figure 2. (a) Close-up of the surgical table in a clinic-based procedure room, holding a single-use tray of sterile instruments, sutures, wound dressing, gauze, Coban wrap, and a water basin. (b) Close-up of sterile instruments included in the single-use instrument tray.

4. Complications and Safety

With the striking changes made to CTR by the use of WALANT, it is important to consider ways in which this could negatively affect outcomes. While complications are possible with any surgical procedure, some practitioners have feared that certain complications are more likely to occur as a result of the nature of WALANT procedures. These complications can be grouped as follows: infection-related complications; bleeding-related complications; and complications stemming from the use of local anesthesia (most commonly, a combination of lidocaine and epinephrine).

4.1. Infections

As discussed, procedures under WALANT are often performed with less extensive sterility set-ups. Thus, it is possible that WALANT could be associated with more surgical site infections. However, no studies to date have demonstrated higher infection rates when WALANT has been used, regardless of operative location, type of sterility used, or composition of personnel present for the procedure [29,30,33,35–39].

4.2. Bleeding

Another potential complication associated with WALANT is increased risk of intra-operative bleeding from the absence of a tourniquet. The use of epinephrine helps limit intra-operative bleeding, though some studies still show an increase in blood loss with CTR under WALANT. It is important, however, to consider the clinical significance and interpretation of the reported increases in such intra-operative bleeding. Sasor et al. found that, on average, only one more milliliter (mL) of blood was lost when CTR was performed under WALANT than when a tourniquet was used (3.28 mL vs. 4.19 mL). Farzam et al. demonstrated that Bier block anesthesia was more likely to be categorized as "bloodless or little blood", whereas all WALANT surgeries were deemed "bloody field, but performable". Saleh et al. found higher bleeding scores among surgeries performed under WALANT, but noted that the bleeding was always controlled by "simply dabbing the incision site" [40–42]. In a meta-analysis of the literature examining the use of a tourniquet, Olaiya et al. concluded that tourniquet use provided no clinically significant benefit but instead, as we will discuss, led to increased post-operative pain [43]. Additionally, Croutzet and Guinand found that patients were able to safely continue use of anticoagulation or anti-platelet medications when undergoing hand surgery under WALANT without being at increased risk of intra-operative bleeding [44].

4.3. Use of Local Anesthesia

Several concerns regarding the use of local anesthesia still exist as barriers to adoption of WALANT for CTR, despite the literature finding that these risks are exceedingly rare. Local-anesthetic systemic toxicity (LAST) is a risk of using local anesthesia which is considered serious and potentially fatal. However, this has not been reported in the literature for CTR under WALANT and there are several strategies that are in common use to prevent this such as the co-administration of epinephrine [45].

The use of epinephrine in the local anesthetic used for WALANT comes with its own set of risks. These can range from minor effects, such as symptoms of an "adrenaline rush" or transient vasovagal symptoms, to more serious catecholamine-induced arrhythmias [39,46]. Farkash et al. monitored heart rhythms during hand procedures under WALANT and did not find any arrhythmogenic properties associated with the local anesthesia used. They concluded that heart monitoring is not needed during these procedures in patients who have no history of arrhythmias [47]. Another potential risk of using epinephrine during WALANT is digital ischemia. While case reports have shown instances of digital ischemia following use of epinephrine in hand surgeries, including CTR, the literature demonstrates the rarity of such cases in the general population [48–50]. Importantly, 20 mL of 1% lidocaine with 1:100,000 epinephrine and 8.4% bicarbonate are often all that is needed for CTR with WALANT (10 mL between the ulnar and median nerves and 10 mL in the subcutaneous tissue under the incision). This falls below the generally accepted maximal dose of lidocaine with epinephrine (seven mg/kg, equating to 50 mL in a 70-kg adult) [51]. Additionally, easy access to phentolamine allows for quick and efficacious reversal of any epinephrine-induced ischemia [52].

5. Pain Control

Pain control in the WALANT technique has been another point of interest. Several studies have found that WALANT is associated with lower or equal levels of pain when compared with tourniquet-utilizing techniques, monitored anesthesia care (MAC), or nerve-block techniques.

5.1. Intra-Operative and Post-Operative Pain Scores

In multiple studies, WALANT was found to be superior to comparison groups in levels of both intra- and post-operative pain (as measured using a visual analogue scale), and of analgesic need. Some studies even went as far as attributing most of the patient's discomfort to the use of a tourniquet [18,41,42,53,54]. Lech et al. focused on patients aged 80 or older and again found significantly less pain post-operatively in the WALANT group than in patients who underwent IV regional anesthesia with a tourniquet [55].

However, the results have not been entirely consistent across studies. While Far-Riera et al. found that the WALANT group had significantly lower levels of post-operative pain, with less analgesic need than comparison groups, they reported similar intra-operative pain across the anesthesia types [56]. Additionally, several studies found no differences in intra- or post-operative pain between WALANT groups, IV regional anesthesia groups, or MAC groups [20,57,58]. Beyond these studies of neutral conclusion, there emerges the possibility that WALANT provides at least an opportunity of decreasing both intra- and post-operative pain experienced by patients, and in many cases leads to decreased observable and reported pain.

5.2. Opioid Use

When WALANT was first introduced, there were concerns that patients would need more analgesia post-operatively since lighter anesthesia was used during the procedure. However, this has not been the finding in studies that have explored this topic. Aultman et al. and Miller et al. found minimal differences in opioid use between the WALANT and MAC cohorts [59,60]. Chapman et al. similarly saw no difference in post-operative consumption of opioids between WALANT and general anesthesia patients, concluding that age and gender were more predictive of opioid consumption than anesthesia type [61]. Kang et al. did, however, observe that there was less need for supplemental opioid injections in the wide-awake group than in the general anesthesia group (12% versus 35%, respectively), showing that there is a strong possibility that WALANT could be beneficial in reducing the need for opioids [62]. Additionally, Dar et al. demonstrated that WALANT patients who were not prescribed opioids following surgery experienced lower pain scores at 14 days post-operation than patients who underwent similar procedures under MAC [63]. This finding suggests that the need for opioid prescriptions post-operatively might be reduced after utilizing the WALANT technique. Further studies would be beneficial in elucidating the possibility that WALANT might decrease opioid use. These initial findings are promising and confirm that the WALANT technique is not associated with increased post-operative analgesia need or use.

6. Return to Functioning

The changes to the standard post-operative course of CTR necessary for the use of WALANT signify that it is possible that patients could have different timelines for returning to function. Thus far, no studies have suggested that returning to function following CTR under WALANT is any worse or takes longer. Thompson Orfeld et al. demonstrated that, following a unilaterally modelled WALANT procedure, patients' driving skills were not negatively impacted. This suggests it could be safe to drive home following a procedure under WALANT, which is not the case with other types of anesthesia [64]. Kang et al. and Iqbal et al. found patients who underwent CTR with WALANT reported similar post-operative functional outcomes as compared with comparison groups who received general anesthesia or wide-awake anesthesia with a tourniquet [62,65]. Interestingly, Karamanis et al. showed that functional outcomes after CTR with WALANT did not differ regardless of the type of local anesthetic used [36].

7. Patient Satisfaction and Perspective

While patient satisfaction with CTR tends to be high, some studies have suggested that patient satisfaction is even higher with CTR performed under WALANT. We credit this to many of the reasons we have previously described. Both Ki Lee et al. and Far-Riera et al. found higher levels of patient-reported satisfaction with CTR under WALANT compared with either local anesthesia with a tourniquet or general anesthesia with a tourniquet [53,56]. Moscato et al. showed that a greater level of satisfaction with WALANT than with other types of anesthesia was consistent across procedural settings [66]. Ayhan took patient perspective a step further and asked patients in both treatment groups to use standard dental procedures for their comparison. Patients in the WALANT cohort were likely to consider CTR dental procedures easier than patients from the IV regional anesthesia group [57]. A handful of studies also showed equivalent relative levels of patient satisfaction between WALANT and comparison groups [20,42,58,59]. Importantly, however, no studies showed decreased levels of patient satisfaction associated with CTR performed under WALANT.

In addition, it is important to consider patients' perspectives and possible anxieties related to undergoing surgery with the WALANT technique. As Morris et al. showed, WALANT offers a solution for patients who are fearful of general anesthesia and its side effects. With regard to WALANT specifically, patients were most concerned with hearing or seeing the procedure as it was being performed and the possibility of feeling pain intra-operatively [67]. Furthermore, Lee et al. found that anxiety was higher among WALANT patients when compared with patients who were given local anesthesia with a tourniquet, although there was no change in overall satisfaction [68]. When compared with general anesthesia, however, Davison et al. reported that the WALANT cohort had significantly less pre-operative anxiety [23].

8. Contraindications to WALANT

While discussing the extensive literature evaluating the use of WALANT for CTR, it is important to clarify circumstances when the WALANT technique is contraindicated. First, it is essential that patients are comfortable with the idea of remaining awake during surgery. As discussed, there are multiple concerns and anxieties that may interfere with the safe execution of CTR under WALANT [67]. It is critical for surgeons to appropriately manage expectations in patients prior to WALANT procedures, as patients with certain comorbidities or low thresholds of anxiety may be better suited to alternative anesthesia methods. Additionally, patients with evidence of peripheral ischemic disease or certain vasculopathies such as scleroderma, Raynaud's disease, Buerger's disease, or a vasculitis could be at increased risk of adverse events from use of local anesthesia. For this reason, it is common for institutions not to offer WALANT to patients with any of the aforementioned conditions [11]. Other conditions that would exclude a patient from WALANT include allergies or hypersensitivities to any component of the local anesthesia that the surgeon plans to use, most often lidocaine and epinephrine [69]. While alternatives to lidocaine have been explored in fields such as dentistry, they have not yet been studied in WALANT. For these scenarios, traditional anesthesia would thus be indicated.

9. Conclusions

As demonstrated in this review of the literature, the WALANT technique for CTR is cost-effective, safe, and patient-centered. Furthermore, its utility and prevalence will continue to grow as health-care systems continue to evolve and greater emphasis is placed on value-based, accessible care.

Author Contributions: Conceptualization, S.M.K.; methodology, K.R.S. and A.D.; writing—original draft preparation, K.R.S. and A.D.; writing—review and editing, K.R.S. and S.M.K.; supervision, S.M.K. All authors have read and agreed to the published version of the manuscript.

Funding: This research received no external funding.

Institutional Review Board Statement: Not applicable.

Informed Consent Statement: Not applicable.

Conflicts of Interest: The authors declare no conflict of interest.

References

1. Atroshi, I.; Gummesson, C.; Johnsson, R.; Ornstein, E.; Ranstam, J.; Rosén, I. Prevalence of carpal tunnel syndrome in a general population. *Jama* **1999**, *282*, 153–158. [CrossRef] [PubMed]
2. Pourmemari, M.-H.; Heliövaara, M.; Viikari-Juntura, E.; Shiri, R. Carpal tunnel release: Lifetime prevalence, annual incidence, and risk factors. *Muscle Nerve* **2018**, *58*, 497–502. [CrossRef] [PubMed]

3. Dale, A.M.; Harris-Adamson, C.; Rempel, D.; Gerr, F.; Hegmann, K.; Silverstein, B.; Burt, S.; Garg, A.; Kapellusch, J.; Merlino, L.; et al. Prevalence and incidence of carpal tunnel syndrome in US working populations: Pooled analysis of six prospective studies. *Scand. J. Work Environ. Health* **2013**, *39*, 495–505. [CrossRef] [PubMed]
4. Feng, B.; Chen, K.; Zhu, X.; Ip, W.Y.; Andersen, L.L.; Page, P.; Wang, Y. Prevalence and risk factors of self-reported wrist and hand symptoms and clinically confirmed carpal tunnel syndrome among office workers in China: A cross-sectional study. *BMC Public Health* **2021**, *21*, 57. [CrossRef]
5. Aboonq, M.S. Pathophysiology of carpal tunnel syndrome. *Neurosciences* **2015**, *20*, 4–9.
6. Kasielska-Trojan, A.; Sitek, A.; Antoszewski, B. Second to fourth digit ratio (2D:4D) in women with carpal tunnel syndrome. *Early Hum. Dev.* **2019**, *137*, 104829. [CrossRef]
7. Fajardo, M.; Kim, S.H.; Szabo, R.M. Incidence of carpal tunnel release: Trends and implications within the United States ambulatory care setting. *J. Hand Surg.* **2012**, *37*, 1599–1605. [CrossRef]
8. Burton, C.L.; Chen, Y.; Chesterton, L.S.; van der Windt, D.A. Trends in the prevalence, incidence and surgical management of carpal tunnel syndrome between 1993 and 2013: An observational analysis of UK primary care records. *BMJ Open* **2018**, *8*, e020166. [CrossRef]
9. Grandizio, L.C.; Graham, J.; Klena, J.C. Current Trends in WALANT Surgery: A Survey of American Society for Surgery of the Hand Members. *J. Hand Surg. Glob. Online* **2020**, *2*, 186–190. [CrossRef]
10. Turcotte, J.J.; Gelfand, J.M.; Jones, C.M.; Jackson, R.S. Development of a Low-Resource Operating Room and a Wide-Awake Orthopedic Surgery Program During the COVID-19 Pandemic. *Surg. Innov.* **2021**, *28*, 183–188. [CrossRef]
11. Kurtzman, J.S.; Etcheson, J.I.; Koehler, S.M. Wide-awake Local Anesthesia with No Tourniquet: An Updated Review. *Plast. Reconstr. Surg. Glob. Open* **2021**, *9*, e3507. [CrossRef] [PubMed]
12. Fnais, N.; Gomes, T.; Mahoney, J.; Alissa, S.; Mamdani, M. Temporal trend of carpal tunnel release surgery: A population-based time series analysis. *PLoS ONE* **2014**, *9*, e97499. [CrossRef] [PubMed]
13. Leblanc, M.R.; Lalonde, J.; Lalonde, D.H. A detailed cost and efficiency analysis of performing carpal tunnel surgery in the main operating room versus the ambulatory setting in Canada. *Hand* **2007**, *2*, 173–178. [CrossRef]
14. Kazmers, N.H.; Presson, A.P.; Xu, Y.; Howenstein, A.; Tyser, A.R. Cost Implications of Varying the Surgical Technique, Surgical Setting, and Anesthesia Type for Carpal Tunnel Release Surgery. *J. Hand Surg.* **2018**, *43*, 971–977.e971. [CrossRef] [PubMed]
15. White, M.; Parikh, H.R.; Wise, K.L.; Vang, S.; Ward, C.M.; Cunningham, B.P. Cost Savings of Carpal Tunnel Release Performed In-Clinic Compared to an Ambulatory Surgery Center: Time-Driven Activity-Based-Costing. *Hand* **2021**, *16*, 746–752. [CrossRef] [PubMed]
16. Chatterjee, A.; McCarthy, J.E.; Montagne, S.A.; Leong, K.; Kerrigan, C.L. A cost, profit, and efficiency analysis of performing carpal tunnel surgery in the operating room versus the clinic setting in the United States. *Ann. Plast. Surg.* **2011**, *66*, 245–248. [CrossRef] [PubMed]
17. Rogers, M.J.; Stephens, A.R.; Yoo, M.; Nelson, R.E.; Kazmers, N.H. Optimizing Costs and Outcomes for Carpal Tunnel Release Surgery: A Cost-Effectiveness Analysis from Societal and Health-Care System Perspectives. *J. Bone Jt. Surg. Am.* **2021**, *103*, 2190–2199. [CrossRef] [PubMed]
18. Okamura, A.; Moraes, V.Y.; Fernandes, M.; Raduan-Neto, J.; Belloti, J.C. WALANT versus intravenous regional anesthesia for carpal tunnel syndrome: A randomized clinical trial. *Sao Paulo Med. J.* **2021**, *139*, 576–578. [CrossRef]
19. Alter, T.H.; Warrender, W.J.; Liss, F.E.; Ilyas, A.M. A Cost Analysis of Carpal Tunnel Release Surgery Performed Wide Awake versus under Sedation. *Plast. Reconstr. Surg.* **2018**, *142*, 1532–1538. [CrossRef]
20. Via, G.G.; Esterle, A.R.; Awan, H.M.; Jain, S.A.; Goyal, K.S. Comparison of Local-Only Anesthesia Versus Sedation in Patients Undergoing Staged Bilateral Carpal Tunnel Release: A Randomized Trial. *Hand* **2020**, *15*, 785–792. [CrossRef]
21. Kamal, R.N.; Behal, R. Clinical Care Redesign to Improve Value in Carpal Tunnel Syndrome: A Before-and-After Implementation Study. *J. Hand Surg.* **2019**, *44*, 1–8. [CrossRef] [PubMed]
22. De Boccard, O.; Müller, C.; Christen, T. Economic impact of anaesthesia methods used in hand surgery: Global costs and operating room's throughput. *J. Plast. Reconstr. Aesthet. Surg.* **2021**, *74*, 2149–2155. [CrossRef] [PubMed]
23. Davison, P.G.; Cobb, T.; Lalonde, D.H. The patient's perspective on carpal tunnel surgery related to the type of anesthesia: A prospective cohort study. *Hand* **2013**, *8*, 47–53. [CrossRef] [PubMed]
24. Rhee, P.C.; Fischer, M.M.; Rhee, L.S.; McMillan, H.; Johnson, A.E. Cost Savings and Patient Experiences of a Clinic-Based, Wide-Awake Hand Surgery Program at a Military Medical Center: A Critical Analysis of the First 100 Procedures. *J. Hand Surg.* **2017**, *42*, e139–e147. [CrossRef] [PubMed]
25. Grimes, C.E.; Bowman, K.G.; Dodgion, C.M.; Lavy, C.B.D. Systematic Review of Barriers to Surgical Care in Low-Income and Middle-Income Countries. *World J. Surg.* **2011**, *35*, 941–950. [CrossRef]
26. Rose, J.; Weiser, T.G.; Hider, P.; Wilson, L.; Gruen, R.L.; Bickler, S.W. Estimated need for surgery worldwide based on prevalence of diseases: A modelling strategy for the WHO Global Health Estimate. *Lancet Glob. Health* **2015**, *3*, S13–S20. [CrossRef]
27. Behar, B.J.; Danso, O.O.; Farhat, B.; Ativor, V.; Abzug, J.; Lalonde, D.H. Collaboration in Outreach: The Kumasi, Ghana, Model. *Hand Clin.* **2019**, *35*, 429–434. [CrossRef]
28. Holoyda, K.A.; Farhat, B.; Lalonde, D.H.; Owusu-Danso, O.; Agbenorku, P.; Hoyte-Williams, P.E.; Rockwell, W.B. Creating an Outpatient, Local Anesthetic Hand Operating Room in a Resource-Constrained Ghanaian Hospital Builds Surgical Capacity and Financial Stability. *Ann. Plast. Surg.* **2020**, *84*, 385–389. [CrossRef]

29. Leblanc, M.R.; Lalonde, D.H.; Thoma, A.; Bell, M.; Wells, N.; Allen, M.; Chang, P.; McKee, D.; Lalonde, J. Is main operating room sterility really necessary in carpal tunnel surgery? A multicenter prospective study of minor procedure room field sterility surgery. *Hand* **2011**, *6*, 60–63. [CrossRef]
30. Avoricani, A.; Dar, Q.-A.; Levy, K.H.; Kurtzman, J.S.; Koehler, S.M. WALANT Hand and Upper Extremity Procedures Performed with Minor Field Sterility Are Associated with Low Infection Rates. *Plast. Surg.* **2022**, *30*, 122–129. [CrossRef]
31. Yu, J.; Ji, T.A.; Craig, M.; McKee, D.; Lalonde, D.H. Evidence-based Sterility: The Evolving Role of Field Sterility in Skin and Minor Hand Surgery. *Plast. Reconstr. Surg. Glob. Open* **2019**, *7*, e2481. [CrossRef] [PubMed]
32. Peters, B.; Giuffre, J.L. Canadian Trends in Carpal Tunnel Surgery. *J. Hand Surg.* **2018**, *43*, e1031–e1035. [CrossRef] [PubMed]
33. Avoricani, A.; Dar, Q.A.; Levy, K.H.; Koehler, S.M. WALANT Hand Surgery: Do the AORN Guidelines Apply? *J. Surg. Orthop. Adv.* **2021**, *30*, 156–160. [PubMed]
34. Maliha, S.G.; Cohen, O.; Jacoby, A.; Sharma, S. A Cost and Efficiency Analysis of the WALANT Technique for the Management of Trigger Finger in a Procedure Room of a Major City Hospital. *Plast. Reconstr. Surg.–Glob. Open* **2019**, *7*, e2509. [CrossRef] [PubMed]
35. Rellán, I.; Bronenberg Victorica, P.; Kohan Fortuna Figueira, S.V.; Donndorff, A.G.; De Carli, P.; Boretto, J.G. What Is the Infection Rate of Carpal Tunnel Syndrome and Trigger Finger Release Performed Under Wide-Awake Anesthesia? *Hand* **2021**, 1558944721994262. [CrossRef] [PubMed]
36. Karamanis, N.; Stamatiou, G.; Vasdeki, D.; Sakellaridis, N.; Xarchas, K.C.; Varitimidis, S.; Dailiana, Z.H. Wide Awake Open Carpal Tunnel Release: The Effect of Local Anesthetics in the Postoperative Outcome. *J. Hand Microsurg.* **2021**, *13*, 95–100. [CrossRef]
37. Randall, D.J.; Peacock, K.; Nickel, K.B.; Olsen, M.; Tyser, A.R.; Kazmers, N.H. Comparison of Complication Risk for Open Carpal Tunnel Release: In-office versus Operating Room Settings. *Plast. Reconstr. Surg. Glob. Open* **2021**, *9*, e3685. [CrossRef]
38. Jagodzinski, N.A.; Ibish, S.; Furniss, D. Surgical site infection after hand surgery outside the operating theatre: A systematic review. *J. Hand Surg. Eur. Vol.* **2017**, *42*, 289–294. [CrossRef]
39. Croutzet, P.; Guinand, R.; Djerbi, I. Birth and Growth of an Ultrasound Hand Surgery Center: A review of 1167 procedures. *Orthop. J. Sports Med.* **2019**, *7*, 2325967119S00216. [CrossRef]
40. Sasor, S.E.; Cook, J.A.; Duquette, S.P.; Lucich, E.A.; Cohen, A.C.; Wooden, W.A.; Tholpady, S.; Chu, M. Tourniquet Use in Wide-Awake Carpal Tunnel Release. *Hand* **2020**, *15*, 59–63. [CrossRef]
41. Farzam, R.; Deilami, M.; Jalili, S.; Kamali, K. Comparison of Anesthesia Results between Wide Awake Local Anesthesia no Tourniquet (WALANT) and Forearm Tourniquet Bier Block in Hand Surgeries: A Randomized Clinical Trial. *Arch. Bone Jt. Surg.* **2021**, *9*, 116–121. [PubMed]
42. Saleh, E.; Saleh, J.; Govshievich, A.; Ferland-Caron, G.; Lin, J.C.; Tremblay, D.M. Comparing Minor Hand Procedures Performed with or without the Use of a Tourniquet: A Randomized Controlled Trial. *Plast. Reconstr. Surg. Glob. Open* **2021**, *9*, e3513. [CrossRef] [PubMed]
43. Olaiya, O.R.; Alagabi, A.M.; Mbuagbaw, L.; McRae, M.H. Carpal Tunnel Release without a Tourniquet: A Systematic Review and Meta-Analysis. *Plast. Reconstr. Surg.* **2020**, *145*, 737–744. [CrossRef] [PubMed]
44. Croutzet, P.; Guinand, R. Maintaining anticoagulant treatment in hand surgery—A review of 63 procedures. *Hand Surg. Rehabil.* **2017**, *36*, 428. [CrossRef]
45. Mulroy, M.F.; Hejtmanek, M.R. Prevention of local anesthetic systemic toxicity. *Reg. Anesth. Pain Med.* **2010**, *35*, 177–180. [CrossRef]
46. Greene, B.H.C.; Lalonde, D.H.; Seal, S.K.F. Incidence of the "Adrenaline Rush" and Vasovagal Response with Local Anesthetic Injection. *Plast. Reconstr. Surg. Glob. Open* **2021**, *9*, e3659. [CrossRef]
47. Farkash, U.; Herman, A.; Kalimian, T.; Segal, O.; Cohen, A.; Laish-Farkash, A. Keeping the Finger on the Pulse: Cardiac Arrhythmias in Hand Surgery Using Local Anesthesia with Adrenaline. *Plast. Reconstr. Surg.* **2020**, *146*, 54e–60e. [CrossRef]
48. Zhu, A.F.; Hood, B.R.; Morris, M.S.; Ozer, K. Delayed-Onset Digital Ischemia After Local Anesthetic with Epinephrine Injection Requiring Phentolamine Reversal. *J. Hand Surg.* **2017**, *42*, e471–e479. [CrossRef]
49. Lalonde, D.; Bell, M.; Benoit, P.; Sparkes, G.; Denkler, K.; Chang, P. A multicenter prospective study of 3110 consecutive cases of elective epinephrine use in the fingers and hand: The Dalhousie Project clinical phase. *J. Hand Surg.* **2005**, *30*, 1061–1067. [CrossRef]
50. Abdullah, S.; Chia Hua, L.; Sheau Yun, L.; Devapitchai, A.S.T.; Ahmad, A.A.; Singh, P.S.G.N.; Sapuan, J. A Review of 1073 Cases of Wide-Awake-Local-Anaesthesia-No-Tourniquet (WALANT) in Finger and Hand Surgeries in an Urban Hospital in Malaysia. *Cureus* **2021**, *13*, e16269. [CrossRef]
51. Lalonde, D.H.; Wong, A. Dosage of local anesthesia in wide awake hand surgery. *J. Hand Surg.* **2013**, *38*, 2025–2028. [CrossRef] [PubMed]
52. Moog, P.; Dozan, M.; Betzl, J.; Sukhova, I.; Kükrek, H.; Megerle, K. WALANT-Epinephrine injection may lead to short term, reversible episodes of critical oxygen saturation in the fingertips. *Arch. Orthop. Trauma. Surg.* **2021**, *141*, 527–533. [CrossRef] [PubMed]
53. Ki Lee, S.; Gul Kim, S.; Sik Choy, W. A randomized controlled trial of minor hand surgeries comparing wide awake local anesthesia no tourniquet and local anesthesia with tourniquet. *Orthop. Traumatol. Surg. Res.* **2020**, *106*, 1645–1651. [CrossRef] [PubMed]

54. Gunasagaran, J.; Sean, E.S.; Shivdas, S.; Amir, S.; Ahmad, T.S. Perceived comfort during minor hand surgeries with wide awake local anaesthesia no tourniquet (WALANT) versus local anaesthesia (LA)/tourniquet. *J. Orthop. Surg.* **2017**, *25*, 2309499017739499. [CrossRef] [PubMed]
55. Lech, L.; Leitsch, S.; Krug, C.; Bonaccio, M.; Haas, E.; Holzbach, T. Open Carpal Tunnel Release Under WALANT—Suitable for All Ages? *J. Hand Surg. Glob. Online* **2021**, *3*, 129–132. [CrossRef] [PubMed]
56. Far-Riera, A.M.; Pérez-Uribarri, C.; Sánchez Jiménez, M.; Esteras Serrano, M.J.; Rapariz González, J.M.; Ruiz Hernández, I.M. Prospective study on the application of a WALANT circuit for surgery of tunnel carpal syndrome and trigger finger. *Rev. Esp. Cir. Ortop. Traumatol.* **2019**, *63*, 400–407.
57. Ayhan, E.; Akaslan, F. Patients' Perspective on Carpal Tunnel Release with WALANT or Intravenous Regional Anesthesia. *Plast. Reconstr. Surg.* **2020**, *145*, 1197–1203. [CrossRef] [PubMed]
58. Tulipan, J.E.; Kim, N.; Abboudi, J.; Liss, F.; Kirkpatrick, W.; Rivlin, M.; Wang, M.L.; Matzon, J.; Ilyas, A.M.; Tulipan, J.E. Open Carpal Tunnel Release Outcomes: Performed Wide Awake versus with Sedation. *J. Hand Microsurg.* **2017**, *9*, 74–79. [PubMed]
59. Aultman, H.; Roth, C.A.; Curran, J.; Angeles, J.; Mass, D.; Wolf, J.M.; Mica, M.C. Prospective Evaluation of Surgical and Anesthetic Technique of Carpal Tunnel Release in an Orthopedic Practice. *J. Hand Surg.* **2021**, *46*, e61–e69. [CrossRef] [PubMed]
60. Miller, A.; Kim, N.; Ilyas, A.M. Prospective Evaluation of Opioid Consumption Following Hand Surgery Performed Wide Awake Versus with Sedation. *Hand* **2017**, *12*, 606–609. [CrossRef]
61. Chapman, T.; Kim, N.; Maltenfort, M.; Ilyas, A.M. Prospective Evaluation of Opioid Consumption Following Carpal Tunnel Release Surgery. *Hand* **2017**, *12*, 39–42. [CrossRef] [PubMed]
62. Kang, S.W.; Park, H.M.; Park, J.K.; Jeong, H.-S.; Cha, J.-K.; Go, B.-S.; Min, K.-T. Open cubital and carpal tunnel release using wide-awake technique: Reduction of postoperative pain. *J. Pain Res.* **2019**, *12*, 2725–2731. [CrossRef]
63. Dar, Q.A.; Avoricani, A.; Rompala, A.; Levy, K.H.; Shah, N.V.; Choueka, D.; White, C.M.; Koehler, S.M. WALANT Hand Surgery Does Not Require Postoperative Opioid Pain Management. *Plast. Reconstr. Surg.* **2021**, *148*, 121–130. [CrossRef] [PubMed]
64. Thompson Orfield, N.J.; Badger, A.E.; Tegge, A.N.; Davoodi, M.; Perez, M.A.; Apel, P.J. Modeled Wide-Awake, Local-Anesthetic, No-Tourniquet Surgical Procedures Do Not Impair Driving Fitness: An Experimental On-Road Noninferiority Study. *J. Bone Jt. Surg. Am.* **2020**, *102*, 1616–1622. [CrossRef] [PubMed]
65. Iqbal, H.J.; Doorgakant, A.; Rehmatullah, N.N.T.; Ramavath, A.L.; Pidikiti, P.; Lipscombe, S. Pain and outcomes of carpal tunnel release under local anaesthetic with or without a tourniquet: A randomized controlled trial. *J. Hand Surg. Eur. Vol.* **2018**, *43*, 808–812. [CrossRef]
66. Moscato, L.; Helmi, A.; Kouyoumdjian, P.; Lalonde, D.; Mares, O. The impact of WALANT anesthesia and office-based settings on patient satisfaction after carpal tunnel release: A patient reported outcome study. *Orthop. Traumatol. Surg. Res.* **2021**, 103134. [CrossRef] [PubMed]
67. Morris, M.T.; Rolf, E.; Tarkunde, Y.R.; Dy, C.J.; Wall, L.B. Patient Concerns About Wide-Awake Local Anesthesia No Tourniquet (WALANT) Hand Surgery. *J. Hand Surg.* **2021**. [CrossRef] [PubMed]
68. Lee, S.K.; Kim, W.S.; Choy, W.S. A randomized controlled trial of three different local anesthetic methods for minor hand surgery. *J. Orthop. Surg.* **2022**, *30*, 23094990211047280. [CrossRef] [PubMed]
69. Jenerowicz, D.; Polańska, A.; Glińska, O.; Czarnecka-Operacz, M.; Schwartz, R.A. Allergy to lidocaine injections: Comparison of patient history with skin testing in five patients. *Postepy Derm. Alergol.* **2014**, *31*, 134–138. [CrossRef] [PubMed]

MDPI
St. Alban-Anlage 66
4052 Basel
Switzerland
Tel. +41 61 683 77 34
Fax +41 61 302 89 18
www.mdpi.com

Journal of Clinical Medicine Editorial Office
E-mail: jcm@mdpi.com
www.mdpi.com/journal/jcm

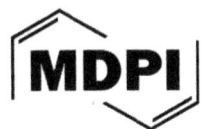

www.ingramcontent.com/pod-product-compliance
Lightning Source LLC
LaVergne TN
LVHW070556100526
838202LV00012B/484